PRAISE FOR *SEX THAT WORKS*

"As a couples therapist who regularly works with clients on issues related to attachment and emotional regulation, I welcome loveologist Wendy Strgar's new book, *Sex That Works*, with its abundance of tools for individuals and couples seeking to improve their emotional and sexual lives. The themes around which the book is organized—freedom, pleasure, courage, curiosity, sensation, attention, and more—are the foundation not only to a satisfying sex life but also to a mutually respectful and secure-functioning relationship."

STAN TATKIN, PSYD, MFT
author of *Wired for Love* and *Wired for Dating*; founder of the PACT Institute

"Wendy Strgar's new book, *Sex That Works*, has captured the struggle: deep within our erotic selves, we all have a desire to be free to pursue sexual pleasure. With her own life and the stories of couples just like us, it is clear that she knows this world. She has lived it; she is an expert in true intimacy. She helps us to express our fantasies through fun and easy-to-understand exercises. Strgar shows us how to find the courage to ask for what we want and reassures us that there is no such thing as 'normal.'"

TAMMY NELSON, PHD
board-certified sexologist; AASECT-certified sex therapist;
author of *Getting the Sex You Want* and *The New Monogamy*

"Erotic bliss is everyone's birthright. The teachings in this book point the way to emotional healing, empowered authenticity, and passion beyond your wildest expectations."

GAY HENDRICKS, PHD
author of the bestselling books
Conscious Loving, *The Big Leap*, and *Five Wishes*

"As a wholistic sexuality teacher, I resonate deeply with loveologist Wendy Strgar's *Sex That Works*. Her wise words offer an insightful and encompassing deep dive into the real sexual arts: connection, feelings, intimacy, communication, and pleasure. Now at the top of my 'must read' list, this book is for anyone who wants to transform their sex lives into a celebration of freedom. You can learn to delight in deeply embodied pleasure, and *Sex That Works* will lovingly guide you on your way!"

SHERI WINSTON
award-winning author of *Women's Anatomy of Arousal* and
Succulent SexCraft; director of the Intimate Arts Center

"Part memoir, part meditation, Wendy Strgar's new book is *all* sex and *all* passion. Pick a page—any page—of *Sex That Works*, and you'll be sure to find a pearl of sexual wisdom."

IAN KERNER, PHD, LMFT
sex therapist and author of *She Comes First*

"Sex is shrouded in so much mystery and secrecy, and considered so personal, that it's a wonder that we can ever have an honest conversation about it. *Sex That Works* provides a remedy for this. Wendy Strgar speaks openly and frankly about what sex is and how we can attain not only its simple physical pleasures, but also a deep understanding of our complex individual sexual 'truth,' in all its manifestations, through our fantasies and desires.

Through well-chosen real-life stories and practical exercises, Strgar demystifies questions and myths that many of us have about sex and teaches us how to allow vulnerability, honor sexual freedom and responsibility, and ultimately attain the sexual courage that leads to authentic and fulfilling sexual relationships.

This is a book that everyone should read. Its lesson would well serve our children and generations that follow in transforming our moralistic, yet sex-obsessed society to one that appreciates the deeper meaning and value of sex."

STANLEY SIEGEL, LCSW
author of *Your Brain on Sex*

"*Sex That Works* is about far more than sex. It's an invitation to connect with your feelings, explore your sexuality, and heal the broken areas that hold us all back from sexual intimacy and connection. Highly recommended reading!"

DEBBY HERBENICK, PHD
associate professor at Indiana University and author of *Because It Feels Good: A Woman's Guide to Sexual Pleasure and Satisfaction*

"Simply put, I love this book! Wendy Strgar invites us to stop repressing ourselves, our senses, our fantasies, our possibilities. She teaches many new steps in the dance of our erotic and sensual lives and illuminates areas to explore to better understand and embrace ourselves, our intimate partners, and to mine the gold of our potential. Let this book awaken you on every level, and it will widen your heart, your mind, your erotic soul, and your life."

BARBARA MUSSER
author of *Sexy After Cancer*

"Wendy Strgar is a genuine pioneer in the important and emerging field of human sexuality. In her new book, she lifts the cultural taboos on the experience of pleasure and the erotic self out of the shadows and into the light. Strgar calls for the eradication of long-standing cultural and personal shame, and she stresses the importance of learning how to feel, and thereby experience, emotional healing and freedom. Strgar provides a brilliant road map out of secrecy and into sexual freedom."

SUSAN TATE
Eugene Energy Medicine in Eugene, OR

SEX *That* WORKS

ALSO BY WENDY STRGAR

Love That Works: A Guide to Enduring Intimacy

SEX *That* WORKS

An Intimate Guide to

Awakening

Your Erotic Life

WENDY STRGAR

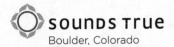

SOUNDS TRUE
Boulder, Colorado

Sounds True
Boulder, CO 80306

Published 2017

Cover design by Lisa Kerans
Book design by Beth Skelley

Printed in Canada

Library of Congress Cataloging-in-Publication Data
Names: Strgar, Wendy, author.
Title: Sex that works : an intimate guide to awakening your erotic life /
    Wendy Strgar.
Description: Boulder, CO : Sounds True, [2017] | Includes bibliographical
    references and index.
Identifiers: LCCN 2016043431 (print) | LCCN 2016059901 (ebook) |
    ISBN 9781622038893 (pbk.) | ISBN 9781622038909 (ebook)
Subjects: LCSH: Sex instruction. | Sexual excitement. | Sexual intercourse.
Classification: LCC HQ31 .S96 2017 (print) | LCC HQ31 (ebook) |
    DDC 613.9/6—dc23
LC record available at https://lccn.loc.gov/2016043431

10 9 8 7 6 5 4 3 2 1

For Franc
and the mystical, healing, wondrous love we make.

And for our children—Emma, Luke, Ian, and Anastasia—
who have taught my heart to feel everything.

The way you make love is the way

God will be with you.

RUMI

CONTENTS

INTRODUCTION

LEARNING TO FEEL

A good friend of mine recently told me that her resolution for this year was to become more human. She laughed as she shared the story of how some of her friends from Silicon Valley didn't quite understand what she meant.

"I am serious," she said. "I want to feel more."

Her desire struck me because in many ways it seems to be the opposite of what we, as a culture, want. Our lives are increasingly dominated by digital gadgets that offer at best a superficial connectivity, though they allow unprecedented productivity. Thanks to technology, we get more done and faster. *Feelings*—who has time for those? And when our relationships begin to fail, when our sex lives disappear, we look for quick fixes—prescriptions for libido, energy enhancers, casual encounters. We search the Internet, when really it is time to begin to look within.

Maybe it's no wonder; learning to feel isn't easy. Feelings are like weather patterns: they are changeable and powerful, and if they reflect the nature of the moment, they can also distract and even frighten us with their intensity. Small children are frequently shaken by the power of their feelings. When was the last time you witnessed a temper tantrum in the grocery store, a giant storm raging inside a little body? What happened when your feelings were too big to hold when you were a child? What could happen if you let yourself experience those feelings now?

Yet our ability to experience and share our feelings in meaningful ways is one of the profound marks of our humanity. Our feelings, as my friend recognized, are what make us human.

One thing that I have learned is that without a capacity to feel, we cannot build or sustain intimate relationships. For the past twelve years, I've been studying love, thinking and writing about sexual intimacy as an integral part of building lasting relationships and sustaining health. Since I study love, *loveologist* is the best name for my occupation. I'm also a successful entrepreneur of love products, which means on the days when I'm not flying on a plane for seven hours to go to a trade show or a sales meeting, I'm in the office wrestling with the everyday challenges of running my business. What isn't part of my official biography is that for a woman in her fifties, I have an amazing, off-the-charts sex life. I've been married to the same man for over thirty years, and the depth and breadth of intimacy that I enjoy with my husband not only has been the concrete in the foundation of my marriage but also the inspiration in all my work.

Getting here was by no means easy for me. I grew up in a violent household, where my father's experience of all emotions was limited to a single expression: anger. His rage toward women exponentially expanded after my parents' devastating divorce, and it was confusing and frightening when this rage was directed at me.

Yet in the midst of all this unpleasantness, I was curious about feelings, as kids often are—especially the intense pleasures I was able to experience with my body. Once, after finding the word *masturbation* in an Ann Landers column, I asked my father what it meant. In his crass New York way, he yelled back, "It means jerking off!"

That was the extent of my sex education at home. It taught me not to ask questions. It would be a long time before I learned to stop associating pleasure with guilt and shame.

My first sexual experiences, in my late teens and early twenties, were with dangerous, destructive men—guys who were, no big surprise, jerk-offs. Looking back, I have no doubt that I would have continued down that dark, destructive path had it not been for the help of a therapist my mother (very uncharacteristically) encouraged me to see. I expect that had I not begun, with the help of my therapist, to articulate and *feel* all of the sadness and anger of my childhood, I would have destroyed myself with men who cared nothing for me. Instead, I had the good fortune to begin the work that has made possible the strong relationship I have with my husband. In fact, all of the loving relationships I now have—with my family, friends, and myself—are possible only because of the work I've done (and am still doing) to learn to feel.

The truth is, the only way to true presence in our lives is through our bodies. This is the lesson I've learned. When we reach that place of true presence, everything, including sex, becomes vivid and interesting. But being truly present also means we continually risk feeling pain. This explains our rampant self-medicating—with pills, food, TV, addictive substances of all kinds; we will do anything to numb ourselves to the unpleasant feelings that are part of being human and fully living in our bodies.

But feelings don't work that way. We can't selectively numb ourselves only to the unpleasant ones. When we choose the route of avoidance and addiction, we end up numbing ourselves to *all* of our feelings, including the desirable ones. For too many people—millions, actually—a satisfying erotic experience is often inaccessible because they have abandoned their capacity to feel.

This book, *Sex That Works*, is about making the choice to live a feeling life, to physically experience the internal storms of living in our bodies and being together with other bodies. It is about understanding our bodies as a source of pleasure and joy. The thing is, our feelings are not just some thought in our head; they are the physical sensations of heartbreak or the churning anxiety in our belly that gets stored in the body with every emotion we refuse to feel. How you habitually relate to your feelings impacts how deeply you experience your body and your sex life. Don't get me wrong: feeling our emotions is not easy, but the alternative is worse. Not feeling cuts us off from the richness of our lives and makes us a stranger to our own sexuality.

The book is organized in nine themed chapters. Each chapter includes stories, skill-building activities, and kernels of wisdom I've gleaned as a loveologist, to help you transfigure your erotic life. Each chapter also includes a little of my own story. It isn't always pretty, but the truth is that the more we share our personal erotic journeys, the more we help other people along their way.

The order of the chapters reflects the themes in my own journey, as well as the journeys of the couples and individuals who have come to me searching for the pleasure they know is locked somewhere in their bodies—if only they could find the key. You might encounter these themes in a different order, and no one order is better than another. You could actually pick up this book and begin with a theme that is most compelling to you.

What you won't find in these chapters is an authoritative voice declaring, "*This* is how you feel." I don't think such an approach works. We are all different people, and we all have different work to do. However, I have found that the themes of the journey are, if not universal, widely experienced.

The journey usually begins with the *freedom* that comes from learning to hold ourselves, to take responsibility for our own emotional and erotic lives. Maybe the thing that pushes us toward this freedom is a wish to no longer be alone—a desire for the kind of loving connection that makes our own feelings real. But really, this first step on the journey is about giving ourselves permission to open a space where we can be who we truly are.

Once we have opened this space of freedom, we begin to experience the *pleasure* that we desire and that it is our innate ability to feel. Pleasure becomes our guide. Yet in order to experience deep, lasting pleasure, we have to be able to feel everything that comes our way. We cannot selectively numb ourselves to only the unpleasant feelings and sensations. If we want to be able to feel the pleasure of being embodied, we also have to be willing to feel the pain. Moreover, we need to educate ourselves and learn to talk about what gives us pleasure, in order to both communicate with our partners and help us explore and shape our own experiences.

As we follow our pleasure and develop our erotic selves, our feelings may be accompanied by doubts, the most vocal of which is often, "Am I *normal?*" We wonder if we are normal to be feeling what we are feeling, desiring what we are desiring. With these doubts comes fear. Feelings are, for many people, sealed within a locked box, and to begin to open that box can be frightening. Certainly this was the case for me.

In a variety of circumstances and for a variety of reasons, we are taught to suppress feelings that aren't "normal," and we learn to silence them so well that the messages they send us through our bodies are not even discernible. This stage of our journey is about observing—observing our own ideas of what is normal, observing the people around us and what's normal for them, and starting to open our eyes to the true range of feelings that we are capable of.

Those suppressed feelings are not as invisible as we might think. They take on a life in our dreams and eventually become diseases in our bodies. Our inability to express them not only cuts us off from our own experience but also limits the connection we feel with the people we love most. If we are to become mature in our sexuality, we need to do more than observe; we need to work through and go beyond our fears. We need to have *courage*. Having the courage to feel and then articulate the full range of emotions that comes with intimate connections is, in fact, the do-or-die work of relationships. It is the fuel for the fire of passion, the air that keeps a relationship breathing, the ground for transformation and growing up. Just as our weaknesses and frailties are intimately connected to our virtues and strengths, the ability to express and feel uncomfortable emotions creates the possibility of discovering the love and passion we want most.

With courage comes the ability to explore our *curiosity*. Earlier in our journey, we learned to follow our pleasure; now we begin to look outside the boundaries we thought we had, to seek out and experiment with new pleasures, to question, to wonder. And we may find that we begin to wake up in more ways than just sexually. The world we live in, our loved ones, our own emotions—everything becomes more interesting when we have the true curiosity and courage to explore it.

With our curiosity awakened, we begin to explore a new awareness of the full, powerful range of *sensation* our bodies are capable of. We stop being dominated by our thoughts, which so often keep us rooted in old habits and stale ways of seeing ourselves and our lives, and we start tuning in to all we are capable of perceiving through our senses when our minds are calm and quiet. When we can actually feel what's happening to us—all the myriad sensations the body is capable of having—the ordinary becomes extraordinary, and we can experience bliss.

At this point in our journey, we are likely feeling more comfortable with our bodies and with ourselves as erotic beings. We can use that comfort, that intimacy and trust we've built within ourselves, to start exploring our interior lives through *fantasy*. Our fantasies guide us along the tantalizing and often blurry boundary between pleasure and pain. Following them, we begin to open our bodies to the wild creations of our minds. And because we have learned to be courageous, we might even begin to share our fantasies with a partner, creating the intense intimacy a passionate sex life needs.

Finally, we begin to witness the power of *attention*. If we let our minds run the litany of habitual thoughts, as they so often do, we will not be able to feel our bodies because we will be distracted by our minds. By mastering our attention, we foster and create the experiences that give us pleasure.

And as we live more fully in our bodies, a deep, visceral feeling of *gratitude* naturally arises. This gratitude is the culmination of each of the other stages, and it renews and replenishes us, so that we can stay present with our feelings through all of our life's joys and challenges.

Learning to feel begins with a choice. When we realize that authentic living demands the maturity to open up to our full experience, as messy as it might be, we choose to learn to do so. Once we can, we have the maturity to be grateful for the life and embodiment that make these pleasures possible. We understand how fleeting all our sensations really are, how brief the time is in which we can experience them, and we start to live the brave, authentic life that is centered on what matters, not what merely distracts.

There are plenty of books out there offering tips or techniques for improving sexual performance. Those books have their place, but it's also important to recognize that although sex is something we do with our bodies, it is not something we do with *just* our bodies. Having good sex, sex that *works*, depends on learning to feel.

I've arranged *Sex That Works* to highlight the themes of the journey while still allowing you the space to make your own observations and discoveries. In each chapter, I've also included some exercises related to the theme, to help you in this work of observing and discovering. I invite you to return to these exercises as often as you like. As you navigate your own journey, think of this book as a network of signposts along the way, pointing you toward yourself: a humanly embodied, sexual being.

You will probably find, as I have, that this journey isn't a linear process. For instance, it wasn't until I was in my forties that I started to let myself explore the erotic fantasies my mind wanted to have when I was aroused. Doing this brought up all sorts of new questions about my normality, and I needed a good deal more courage before I was comfortable giving my curiosity free reign and my body space in which to feel the pleasurable sensations of these fantasies. So, rather than a line, think of this journey as a spiral: from time to time you'll pass signposts you've seen before. Luckily, they're still there to guide you. Since you also have the benefit of accruing practice and experience, the challenges start to seem familiar and less daunting.

Learning to feel is a practice, no different than learning a musical instrument. Some days you hit the right notes; other days there is no melody at all. But just by agreeing to the practice, you open yourself up to an intimacy that deepens your connection with yourself, your partner, and your life. It is an intimate journey that makes sex work.

FREEDOM

The beginning of any journey is imbued with an urgency for more freedom—the freedom to know and understand more of who we are. When it comes to creating a sexual life that works, we must begin by understanding and defining our *own* sexual freedom. We cannot have sex that works until we create a space for our own sexual freedom. But that doesn't mean sexual exploits, and it doesn't mean drowning our need for real human connection in a sea of casual hookups.

Sexual freedom is really about responsibility. Yet how many of us truly realize this, even as adults? In my experience, not many.

In this chapter, we'll explore some of the ways we misunderstand what it means to be sexually free and sacrifice our tender, emerging erotic selves for what turn out to be sexual exploits instead of the true freedom we innately crave. I'll also present a few avenues that lead toward healing as well as helpful reminders as you set off on your own journey toward reclaiming your sexual freedom.

A lot of us are still working with a misunderstood notion of sexual freedom. While we understand that "being adult" is synonymous with "being responsible," when it comes to sex, we often lose sight of this vital connection. Especially as young adults, we think being sexually free means acting on impulse, without reflecting on how our actions will impact ourselves and others. How did we get this notion? The confusion starts early. For many of us, it begins during our adolescence, when our emerging erotic identity and newfound sexual desires create deep conflicts with the family and culture we grow up in.

The ideal of sexual freedom is enticing, especially in the years of our earliest sexual development. During adolescence, as many girls contemplate the big moment of losing their virginity, the questions of *when* and *with whom* dominate their thinking. For teen boys, the "first time" is a marker on the road to manhood and is fundamental to how they come to grips with what it means to be male. As this adolescent erotic consciousness emerges, though, it collides with a culture that has segregated sexuality from real human relationships and made it something to objectify, fetishize, and shame. As a consequence, many of us end up misunderstanding sexual *freedom* as *license* to do whatever comes into our heads, whatever we think might give us a little power over this sexuality that we don't understand and aren't allowed to talk about. The ideal of freedom flips on its head, and we find ourselves falling down the slippery slope of sexual irresponsibility.

This transition was no different for me. I was elated to finally have a boyfriend I wanted to "do it" with, but my first time, in the back of a car, was both brief and painful, leaving me wondering what everyone was making such a big deal about. His breaking up with me a few weeks later added a dose of humiliation, which his crazy ex-girlfriend magnified by spray-painting my white car with profanities.

It isn't surprising that I followed this pitiful first time with increasingly desperate grabs at sexual "freedom." I would meet guys in bars, using a fake ID to get in. The sex was painful, and the interactions with guys who couldn't care less about me made me feel increasingly damaged—distanced from myself and afraid to look at how I actually felt. Yet the worse I thought of myself, the more desperate I became to find the loving, intimate connection that I thought sex was supposed to be about. As a child I was easily orgasmic, but this capacity left me entirely during this time. In the name of sexual freedom, I was eroding my ability to trust myself erotically—which, ironically, made me less and less free.

I hit rock bottom during my second year of college after a "relationship" with the social director of my campus's "animal house" fraternity. By the time it ended, I was a wreck—physically, mentally, and emotionally. I couldn't even go back to school.

These experiments in sexual freedom were a far cry from the romantic stories that filled my adolescence. Growing up in a desolate landscape where nobody really showed up for me, at home or anywhere else, I would listen over and over to Barry Manilow's "Ready to Take a Chance Again," longing profoundly for a loving relationship that would hold me and nourish me. It was only years later, after I had crashed and burned in college and had to figure out how to put my emotional life back together, that I learned that being sexually free meant, first and foremost, *being able to hold myself.* Seeking solace from strangers in bars was a dead end. The only person who could give me the freedom I craved was myself.

Even though some things have changed dramatically since then, I don't believe that the experience of a young woman using a hookup app today is much different from my own. I projected my longing for the intimacy and connection of a sexual encounter onto a Barry Manilow song; a young woman today might project the same longing into the vast outlets of social networking. The damage we inflict on our fragile erotic selves is the same, and it is real.

Hitting bottom during college was an important turning point for me. Finally, I started to have an inkling of how I might have misperceived this notion of freedom. I started to see that my actions had real consequences and that what I was doing in the name of sexual freedom didn't feel like freedom at all—instead, what I was doing was another way I betrayed and hurt myself. I wasn't looking out for myself, and the guys I was with certainly weren't looking out for me. Now I think of the end of my freshman year as the beginning of what has become my life's journey of rehabilitating my fragile erotic self and my misconstrued ideals about freedom, especially about sex.

The most important realization I've had is that sexual freedom is intimately, integrally connected to *responsibility*; there really can't be one without the other.

True sexual freedom does not come from acting out; it is not about sexual license. Authentic sexual freedom means taking responsibility for our own sexual needs. It means moving beyond sexual anxiety and damage through education, gaining not only the courage to take ownership of our erotic preferences but also the skills to engage in sexual behavior that is consistently pleasurable. It means growing up sexually and becoming adults. While we understand that "being adult" is synonymous with "being responsible," when it comes to sex, we often lose sight of this vital connection.

Adults are not waiting for someone else to make them feel sexy or give them permission to explore the range of their sexual function; they are comfortable in themselves, comfortable making their own decisions, and comfortable being who they really are. That's true freedom. This kind of freedom, incidentally, also allows them to be truly responsive to the sexual needs of others, which makes them attractive partners—who tend to stay partnered.

Without understanding the vital connection between sexual freedom and personal responsibility, we can never reach the level of sexual maturity where we connect authentically and intimately with others. And without ever having these intimate connections, we cannot experience the full range of our feelings, including the amazing pleasure sensations our bodies are capable of having.

Taking responsibility for ourselves is the piece that most of us completely miss in our youth and often don't discover until we have done significant damage to our erotic souls. It is such an elusive lesson in part because of the cultural silence and shame surrounding the way we think about sex. For many, the sexual education we receive at school and home is as good as a locked box; it gives us few resources and none of the understanding we seek. During our early sexual years, we move through the shadows, trying to make sense of what we are feeling before, during, and after our sexual encounters. Once we're older, we bristle at the idea of honest conversations about sex even between partners, let alone with our children.

Instead, we replace the education and witnessing that we really need to grow into our freedom with our mistaken notion that being free means baring all. We tweet and post about our exploits as a means of feeling them, letting an imagined audience's reaction to us be a proxy for our own sense of self-worth and covering up the devastating impacts of giving our sexual selves away for nothing.

Although I like to think that when it comes to sex education my four kids have had it better than many—their mom, after all, works as a sex educator—I know that each has struggled in their own way to map for themselves the terrain of their sexual freedom. Adding to their difficulties is the Internet culture they've grown up in, with its myriad channels for broadcasting far and wide each and every life event, amplifying the peer pressure to speak, dress, and behave in certain ways. Feeling this pressure, one of my sons had his first sexual encounter in high school with a girl he barely knew, whom he didn't care for, and who didn't care for him, just so he could say he "did it" and escape the stigma of being a virgin.

People have long been obsessed with virginity—whether it should or shouldn't be "lost" and when and how to lose it. Much of our obsession has to do with the shame that always seems to be cloaking sex and sexuality, and so part of waking up to our sexual freedom is removing this cloak. In doing so, we help to create more openness around sex in a world where even the adults don't know how to have mature conversations about their feelings or their bodies. Sexuality is absolutely fundamental to who we are as human beings, yet so many of us don't even know how to begin to talk about it—and if we do try, we end up feeling embarrassed. As a result, the places where our sexuality is damaged, as individuals and as a society, are never brought to light, which only makes the damage more destructive.

Our aberrant denial of what it means to be human and sexual creates strange and harmful behaviors. It was only about a hundred years ago that boys—these would have been our grandfathers and great-grandfathers—could be forced to wear a ring with sharp metal prongs around their penis, which would gouge the penis when it became engorged as a result of a boy's "impure" thoughts or even dreams. We might like to think we've become more accepting since then, but have we? There are plenty of examples of how convoluted our relationship to sex still is. Consider this: we now live in a world where *millions* of girls have had their clitoris brutally removed.[1] Often they are made to undergo this torture by *their own mothers*, who had to undergo it themselves. It seems unimaginable, yet we pass on our own sexual damage to our children—and as a result, we all suffer.

Closer to home for many of us is the epidemic of rape and sexual assault on U.S. college campuses.[2] This is another example of how a damaged relationship to sex is afflicting us all, but especially young people, who are grappling with impaired notions of freedom they've inherited from a culture with a twisted relationship to sex. For many of today's young adults, the current practice of casual hookups through online dating sites is accepted as a normal, even inevitable, part of dating. I have met many beautiful, intelligent young women who routinely have casual sex with strangers they've barely met—and I stress to them that "meeting someone" is not the same as perusing their online profile. Sadly, they believe this is the only way to find someone to be intimate with. Many of these girls, too, have misperceived—as I did—what it means to be sexually free. Not only does this casual sex rarely end in orgasmic pleasure, but also early and persistent damage to our erotic consciousness often leaves us unable to feel at all. I have wondered whether there is a direct connection between the rising number of young people who engage in self-harm and those who have hookup sex.[3]

There is also the recent trend of successful young women being publicly shamed when naked photos of them are posted on the Internet. When actor Jennifer Lawrence's phone was hacked and photos she'd sent to her boyfriend appeared online, she said of the people who had done it, "I just can't imagine being that detached from humanity. I can't imagine being that thoughtless and careless and so empty inside."[4] A number of other female celebrities also received threats, saying they would be next, from the same people. We can all see the double standard here: these are women who might be expected to pose nude onscreen, where their naked sexuality can be accepted because it is distanced from reality by the trappings of Hollywood, but when they appear naked outside that context, it's assumed they will be shamed and their reputations ruined.

Genital mutilation, college rapes and sexual assault, hookup culture, photo scandals—these are all symptoms of the same disease: fear and denial of what it means to be human and sexual.

The problem is made even more convoluted, especially in the United States, by the prevalence of sexual dysfunction. It impacts nearly half of all women at some point in their lives and typically begins with vaginal dryness, pain with penetration, and an inability to orgasm. Almost as many men deal with premature ejaculation or an inability to have or maintain an erection, as well as generalized anxiety around being sexual. Although our bodies are just as capable of experiencing intense pleasure as they are of experiencing discomfort, for many of us, our early experiences with sex lead us not to pleasure and developing a growing confidence with our sexual maturity, but to suffering and stalled sexual development.

My point in telling you all this bad news is not to be grim but to illustrate that this work of rehabilitating our understanding of sexual freedom is hard and has high stakes. Yet it is the work that will cure the disease of denial and shame around sex.

Waking up sexually starts with breaking the societal barriers that silence our questions and desires. Especially with the people we trust most deeply, we deserve to dare ourselves to wake up to the sexual beings we are.

Our journey of erotic awakening begins with responsibility, and a key part of taking responsibility for your erotic self is recognizing that no one else but you can heal it or make it work. For each of us, the process will look different, because we have each been damaged in different ways.

Yet we are all similar in an important way: we all live in a human body capable of feeling a wide range of painful and pleasant sensations. Sensation—this common, shared space of embodiment—is where we can begin our healing.

For myself, working with sensation—touch, taste, smell, sight, and hearing—has been the key to unlocking my sexuality and all its pleasures. I'll say more about sensation and pleasure in later chapters, but I mention these topics here to show you something bigger than my own story: the process of creating a space of erotic freedom involves practicing, learning, exploring.

To begin our journey toward becoming mature sexual beings, we need to *educate* ourselves about our bodies and our sexuality, and we need to build a vocabulary with which to talk about sex. Education is essential because, just as in other areas of cognition, what we don't know about our sexuality or don't have language to describe disappears from our conscious experience, where we can engage with it rationally. Instead, this ignorance slips into our subconscious, where it impacts our thoughts and bodies even more deeply, but where we have much less access to it—and therefore less ability to transform it.

For example, consider the largely unknown anatomical structure of the internal clitoral erectile network. Contrary to popular belief, the clitoris is not just a small button that sits on top of the vagina; the external glans, containing over 8,000 nerve endings and connected to 15,000 more throughout the pelvis, is the proverbial tip of the iceberg. In fact, the clitoral organ structure closely resembles the male sexual structure, but with long legs that reach deep into the vagina.

It wasn't until the 1990s that research was done which elevated the clitoris to a full organ system that is part of a complex internal erectile network, and not until 2011 did we have an accurate sonographic image. Yet even today, most women have yet to fully understand how to access this complex and profound organ system they are carrying around. One of the researchers, Dr. Pierre Foldès, noted that this internal organ system only functions at its full potential for women who know it is there and are working at cultivating their sensitivity. Knowing about this important network of erectile nerves makes it more possible to experience all of its sensations—thus the long-standing arguments about the existence of the G-spot.[5]

Our lack of knowledge about our sexual selves and the complexity of our sexual functioning is not limited to our anatomy. While pain with sex is almost more common than not, we often know little about its potential causes. And it is the utter silence—and discomfort about breaking our silence—that keeps us locked away from the healing sexual capacity that lives in each of us. The solution to almost all sexual dysfunction begins with open dialogue, not suppression, and to start and maintain this dialogue, we need to educate ourselves.

>> As your first step toward sexual freedom, build a curriculum for yourself and the people you love that allows you to expand your ideas about sexuality and to experience pleasure without shame. This may well mean providing yourself with the sex education you really should have been offered when you were first emerging as an erotic being. A good place to begin is by asking questions and finding the resources and people to help you answer them. You could start with this book's "Further Reading and Resources" section, where I've included some of the resources I've found most helpful.

One thing you can try right now: Make a list of three or four questions you have always had about your own sexual response but never had the nerve to ask anyone. Allow yourself the freedom to ask anything. Don't be surprised if your questions are linked to your deepest fears about your ability to perform or respond sexually. Your questions are the keys to learning that you have needed.

Once you have your questions down, commit to getting real answers. You could do this anonymously by posting on question-and-answer sites such as

Kinsey Confidential, by reading books that will give you insight, or by committing to seeing a sexual health counselor (see "Further Reading and Resources" for where to find one).

You can't find answers to questions you won't ask. Start here and now by asking.

The next step in becoming truly sexually free is to give yourself permission—permission to be curious about your erotic capacity, to explore your body, to experience the mental abandon that is necessary for passionate sex.

So much about our sexual experience is connected to our ability to give ourselves permission to explore the far reaches of arousal. The permission that I am referring to is not deliberative "thinking through the consequences." It is more a visceral form of openness that allows all of the mysterious and hard-to-articulate intensity of sexuality to move through you. We are inherently sexual beings, and this instinctive procreative urge has the power to transform all aspects of our health. By giving ourselves permission to engage fully with all our senses, we call our minds back into our bodies from wherever they may have wandered to during our day's work, and we begin to feel what's happening right here, where we really live—in bodies that are highly sensitive, in living organisms filled with feelings and desires.

No one is exempt from nagging shame and insecurity when they dive deep into their sexuality. But the transcendent emerges from the physical; passion has to replace our more organized, linear thought process in order for our capacity for pleasure to lead us into incredible experiences, the sort we can't believe we've had even moments after having them.

What keeps people from this pleasure delirium is an inability to open up while relinquishing control. Pleasure and passion can seem frightening and unpredictable, especially if you prefer a more controlled and predictable life. For example, think of the leap that has to occur for the couple that thinks sharing a toothbrush is gross to be able to fall headfirst into passionate oral sex. For many people, giving their partner oral sex is simply providing a service. They can't find the pleasure in it, partly because they are not able to give themselves permission to experience the many unpredictable feelings that may arise when you open up to feeling pleasure while giving oral sex.

When I was in the midst of offering myself this permission, I realized that allowing this opening was a close relation to sexual forgiveness. Giving yourself permission to experience pleasure unexpectedly is a way of forgiving yourself. And there is a lot of forgiving that needs to happen around sexuality for most people. Whether from unhelpful cultural messages about what our sexuality means about us or the bad choices most of us made on the way to figuring out our sexuality, we live within a wounded culture of sex that swings wildly between the prudish "just say no" and the casual hookup.

Forgiving ourselves for these choices and loving the wounded places within us is perhaps the most essential commitment we can make when we are permitting ourselves sexual freedom. The more forgiving and accepting we are about our own sexual wounds, the more we can allow our own pleasure, and even more deeply, we can give our partner that same freedom.

And, finally, know this: you are what you love, not what loves you back. This is a profoundly freeing recognition that allows us to experience the depth and breadth of our capacity for love. It is a revolution for the heart to open up to love, the most instructive emotional experience we are capable of having, without hesitation and without worrying about whether our love will be reciprocated. Love teaches without the need for reciprocity, and an understanding of our true selves and our innate freedom develops in us alongside our capacity to give and receive love. No one can take this capacity from us.

>> Practice forgiving yourself. Throughout the day, when you find yourself blaming yourself or being judgmental about who you are, just notice the harsh tone of your inner voice. Listening to how we talk to

ourselves is a way to both befriend our fears and the judgments we hold about ourselves and to interrupt the process so we can replace that negative self-talk with something more helpful.

Just by beginning to notice the moments of negative self-talk, you will be creating more space for a new and forgiving response to emerge. By listening and paying attention to the way you talk to yourself, you increase the chances of speaking to yourself with kindness and acceptance. This takes practice but gets easier the more you do it.

My own route to sexual freedom has taken me a long way from my early days, when I understood sex only in terms of license, exploits, and pain. Now I can say, unabashedly and without hesitation, that I love sex, and it continues to be the most healing and profound area of growth in my life. Establishing authentic sexual freedom in your life makes you more of yourself. Taking responsibility is where we begin to feel we have real control over our sexual evolution. And truly there is nothing else in life that eclipses the culmination of release, joy, and satisfaction I experience each and every time I make love.

I will go further and say that my sex life saves me, restores me to my better self, each and every time I open to it. This is not a minor statement for a woman in her fifties who has been making love to the same man for over thirty years. In fact, it flies in the face of a good deal of current literature on the topic of sexual satisfaction and long-term relationships. Yet here I am, living proof that sex with the same partner over decades can get better and better if it is based on a relationship of true erotic freedom. This truth of this is both one of my best qualifications for my chosen profession and my driving force in trying to spread the word about love. I know from first-hand experience—every week, and if I am lucky, twice a week—that amazing sexual connection is most valuable when it comes to almost any measure of life satisfaction.

You can spot from miles away the couples who have given up on their sex lives. Many of my closest friends' marriages are sexually lonely ones. There is a hardness between the partners, a disappointment that is palpable, even if no one will talk about it out loud. There might not be a lonelier feeling than that of being sexually disconnected from our partner. The truth is I don't know many couples who stay together after they've given up on their sex lives. A dead sex life is the number one reason cited for the dissolution of a relationship.

There is a bonding that happens in physical union. What keeps this bond strong is our experience of erotic freedom within a maturing relationship. And the extravagance of the acts that come out of this erotic freedom is as profound as the tenacity of the bond itself. At the remarkable place where we fully come to our senses and completely forget our egoic self, our erotic capacity is unleashed. It is where we are most animal and also so completely human. The idea that we must lose this space of intellectual abandon and emotional freedom to the familiar confines of long-term relationships is a tragic and, I believe, false conclusion—but one that we keep clinging to. I often hear comments like, "How could I do that with him, when I sit at the table with him every night?" and "How could I do that to her, when she is the mother of my children?"

We have little experience and even less cultural education to help us reconcile the wild in us with our accustomed roles. Yet when we lose our erotic nerve with the people who most intimately inhabit our lives, we are left with little choice but to solicit illicit relationships to discover and reveal our erotic selves. Then, instead of our intimate relationships reveling in the amazing elasticity and strength that provocative eroticism and wild sex contribute to our lives together, we are stuck with the shame of betrayals and a longing for sexual recognition that is always just out of reach.

It isn't like this dichotomy between my sex-crazed self and the woman cooking dinner is lost on me. Coming up for air after the increasingly risqué and surprising sexual acrobatics that my sex life with my husband of thirty years involves often has me at a loss. We lie entwined in the dim candlelight, without words to process what we just did together. And then, after a time, one of us gets up, and quietly we slip back into the middle-aged, long-married parents of four, weighing our options of salad and sardines or going out for take-out.

2

Pleasure

I t is in all of our natures to seek pleasure. When we talk about pleasure, and especially when we talk about the pleasure of good sex, we are not talking about something we do just for fun or something that we should forget about whenever we have more important things to do. We are not talking about a luxury. Sexual pleasure is an essential part of who we are as human beings.

In fact, there is no other activity that carries the physical, mental, and emotional benefits of pleasurable sexual intimacy. A 2004 study by economists at Dartmouth College and the University of Warwick, involving more than 16,000 participants, found that sexual pleasure "enters so strongly [and] positively in happiness equations" that for the average American, increasing intercourse from once a month to once a week generates the same amount of happiness as getting an additional $50,000 in income. The economists calculated that a lasting relationship equates to the happiness that would be generated by getting an extra $100,000 each year. Divorce, meanwhile, translates to a happiness depletion of $66,000 annually.[1]

Hundreds of major medical studies have proven the physical benefits of sex. These studies suggest that an active sex life may lead to a longer lifespan, better heart health, a healthier immune response, reduction in chronic pain symptoms, lower rates of depression, and even protection against some cancers. Lovemaking is also an excellent form of aerobic exercise: it raises your heart rate, engages your muscles, and can lower blood pressure.[2] Studies show that men who have sex twice per week have half as many heart attacks than men who have sex only once per month.[3] Regular sex has been shown to extend the lifespan.[4] In addition, sexual activity dulls the chronic pain of migraines, arthritis, and back pain.[5] A strong sex life will also ease your reactivity to stress, keeping your blood pressure in check when the unexpected happens.[6] And sexually active people are significantly less vulnerable to depression and suicide.[7]

What all of these studies show is that sex feels good *because it is good for us*. Our collective urge to seek pleasure is perhaps the healthiest distinguishing aspect of the gift of our humanity. This is the reason we can use pleasure as a guide to lead us deeper into our erotic selves. Once we have won our erotic freedom, what do we do with it? The answer will come from listening to our sense of pleasure.

When you were a kid, nobody had to teach you how to play. Even the most serious street games of Capture the Flag were fueled by your natural eagerness to move your body, to do what felt good. Having fun was second nature; doing what felt good came automatically. Your youthful spontaneity rode on the tails of the abandon and freedom that came from not worrying about how you were being seen. As we grow up, we seem to forget how important pleasure is to us, how valuable a guide it is to our real feelings. It becomes more difficult to hear the voice of pleasure.

In my own journey, it was the discovery of real pleasure that saved me and my erotic soul. While I was living abroad in France in my twenties, I had an affair with an older man named Michel. After the loneliness and damage of my earlier years, this affair was a bolt of pleasure that awakened my erotic potential, teaching me to access and celebrate my capacity for sexual delight. He craved my sexual energy, and I, for the first time, felt the power and confidence that opening to pleasure provides. As I became bolder as an erotic being, I realized that seeking pleasure was part of my truest nature and that surrendering to its ways was healing.

What I learned from Michel was the importance of understanding and articulating my own pleasure response. He wanted to know what I wanted, and he coaxed me to give words to what touch I liked or didn't. He was patient and inventive. He made me wait and stopped me from rushing toward what I already knew. Sounds simple enough, but at the time, this was a revelation. I found that I was sexy to myself when I was discovering what I liked, and I was even sexier when I was willing to talk about my discoveries. Michel helped me begin to reclaim my erotic voice.

Early in my marriage, before I had fully figured out how I like to be touched and still kept expecting my husband to read my mind, sex always seemed to lead to arguments and hostility. Because I didn't have the language to communicate what I wanted, and he didn't know where his edge was, he would ejaculate prematurely. The rare times we were able to orgasm together, I was equally ecstatic and mystified. I didn't know how we had done it. And the next time we had sex, it was unlikely we would be able to replicate it. Sex, whether it worked or didn't, felt like a locked box that I got to peek into but could never really open.

We were stuck in a situation that many couples find themselves in. In a relationship, communication is like oxygen: it is the air we breathe. Without it, we suffocate, and the relationship withers and dies.

If you have no language for what pleasure is for you, you won't experience much pleasure—or, if you do, it will be a happy accident that you won't be able to reliably replicate. In a relationship, this can lead to all sorts of conflicts around sex—conflicts that make us want to give up on relationships. When it seems like we cannot even be intimate together, then why stay in the relationship? I have encountered so many marriages on the verge of collapse because sex was a site of blame and unarticulated desires and hostilities.

This situation arises because we turn off the voice of our own pleasure. We don't take any responsibility for discovering and communicating what makes us feel good, and then when we aren't immediately satisfied with our sex lives, we blame our partners. The less you are in touch with your own pleasure response, the more dependent you are on someone else to give you pleasure. This dependency is unfair to you, because it keeps you from experiencing all the pleasure that you are really capable of. It is also unfair to your partner, because your pleasure is not really anyone else's responsibility. And it is unfair to your relationship, because an arrangement in which one person is dependent on another is never truly strong and stable.

Sometimes, too, when pleasure seems mysterious and unreliable, and we have no other language with which to comprehend it, we start to attach pleasurable experiences to objects. We develop fetishes, which can be healthy when they enhance or deepen our pleasure, but not when we rely on them so much that we lose touch with our own erotic awareness. Consider a twenty-something couple that can have passionate sex only when both are a little (or a lot) drunk. They come to believe that without alcohol, they cannot have good sex. Because they do not have the language for what is happening in their bodies, they can only see the experience blurrily, without the granularity of apprehension that would show them it isn't the alcohol per se but the relaxing of inhibitions they associate with alcohol that makes the sex so good sometimes. When I discovered the bottle of love oil that released a torrent of passion in my marriage, I developed something of a fetish around that oil. I came to feel that without the oil, I could not have passionate sex. I attached the passion to the oil and not to what was happening in my own mind and body.

The truth is, you cannot hold anyone or anything responsible for your capacity to experience pleasure. When you do, you cheat yourself out of understanding important aspects of yourself. Remaining inarticulate about how you like to be touched, about what feels good for you and what just doesn't work, is like depriving yourself of air or nutrition. It keeps you from growing and maturing, from living fully and wholly. Not only that—it also weakens your relationship with your partner. Fortunately, the opposite is also true: uncovering the keys to your pleasure is empowering and allows you the freedom and courage to open up with a partner in new ways.

>> Remember that playful feeling that came so easily when you were a kid? Treating your quest for more satisfying sex with this same playful, pleasure-seeking spirit can help free your imagination. When we're playful, we don't think in terms of right and wrong, though we do maintain a distinction between fair and unfair. Sexually speaking, being able to play fair and yet play with abandon is the ideal scenario for blossoming into our true erotic selves. But part of playing fair is being responsible for listening to your own pleasure and telling your partner what makes you feel good. With a spirit of playfulness in bed, we can have fun pushing the edges of our comfort zone and know that no matter how it comes out, we will laugh and strengthen our ability to be in the game.

For many of us, taking responsibility for our own pleasure begins with healing our relationship with our body. We may think that we can experience true pleasure only when we look a certain way. *When I lose ten more pounds, I'll deserve a little pleasure. If my tan gets a little deeper, then I'll really be able to feel good.*

Actually, the reverse is true: opening yourself up to more sexual pleasure will make you recognize the beauty in your body as it is and inspire you to treat it better. And here's the thing: if you sacrifice your access to pleasure to the false belief that sexual satisfaction will find you when you are fitter or more beautiful, you will miss out on your own life. Make a decision *now* to stop comparing yourself to the myriad Photoshopped images of models that even models don't look like. Instead, dedicate yourself *now* to finding ways to live more deeply in your body. Sex is something you do with your body, so how you feel about and treat your body is a direct reflection of the respect you hold for your sex life. Resolve to treat your body with a little more attention and loving kindness, and it will reward you by revealing its capacity for pleasure—sexual and otherwise.

If your body needs coaxing, there is something very simple you can do to deepen your relationship with it and explore your pleasure response: masturbate. Even with all the benefits masturbation can bring to a couple's sex life, it is still a behavior that many people are not comfortable sharing with their partners or even talking about. In addition to the religious condemnation that has long been associated with self-pleasure, the practice was not long ago considered an affliction that medical doctors used the cruelest of instruments and techniques to control. So it's not surprising that self-reporting of this behavior still hovers at 30 to 70 percent, depending on gender and age.[8]

Yet there are many benefits to a healthy dose of solo sex. First and foremost, it teaches us about our own sexual response, and personal experience is an invaluable aid when communicating with our partner about what feels good and what doesn't. The practice of solo sex is helpful for men who have issues with premature ejaculation, as it familiarizes them with the moment of inevitability so that they can better master their sense of control. Masturbation can also be a great balancer for couples with a disparity in their sex drive, and solo orgasm can serve as a stress reliever and sleep aid just as well as partnered pleasure can. A 2007 study in *Sexual and Relationship Therapy* reported that male masturbation might also improve immune system functioning and the health of the prostate.[9] For women, it builds pelvic floor muscles and sensitivity and has been associated with reduced back pain and cramping around menses, as it increases blood flow and stimulates relaxation of the area after orgasm.[10]

The one caveat is that masturbation, like anything else, serves us well in moderation. Becoming too obsessed with solo sex play, often enhanced by visual or digital aids, has been known to backfire and lead to loss of interest in the complexity and intensity of partner sex. There are also some forms of masturbation that can make partner sex seem less appealing because the form of self-stimulation is so different from what happens in the paired experience. If you are experiencing less desire or ability to respond to your partner, ask yourself what you can do to make your solo experience more compatible with your partner's ability to stimulate you.

As you become more experienced with the rich and varied pleasures available in your own body and more comfortable communicating your desires to your partner, you may find that there are some experiences you simply don't understand or can't find the right words for. This is normal, and it doesn't mean that you are stupid. It just means that the world we live in sometimes makes it hard for us to educate ourselves about our own bodies and experiences. Many of us lack the knowledge that we need to understand them.

I was forty-seven, believed myself to be sexually open-minded and educated, and had been selling love products for years before I learned about the remarkable clitoral organ system and the complex anatomic structures that rock my inner world every time I orgasm. I am not alone in never having gotten a full tour and understanding of the complex neural network and the multiple organs that work in concert to make sexual pleasure the amazing symphony of sensation that it is. Until about ten years ago, with the advent of books like *The Clitoral Truth* by Rebecca Chalker, much of female anatomy was not understood or taught, even by physicians. Couple this lack of information with a lingering fear of looking at and exploring our private parts, and it is easy to see how so many women have had so little access to or experience with their pleasure centers.

Fortunately, all the knowledge you need is out there, and it is increasingly easy to find if you go looking. The Internet and any of a number of excellent books (some of my favorites are in the "Further Reading and Resources" section at the end of this book) offer insights into your pleasure potential that you never imagined. But the real payoff in this material is that it helps you develop the language to talk about your body. Building a working vocabulary for your most intimate physiology is foundational to developing the capacity to express what feels good when, how, and where. Acquiring the terms that define the physiology of the visible vaginal parts—the mons, labia major and minor, and the clitoral head and hood—is also the starting point to fully grasping the erectile wonders of those same body parts and their connection to the complex internal organs they arouse.

As you learn more, it helps to notice how the language you are already using around sex can keep you from the connection and pleasure you want. For instance, joking about genitalia may be accept-able among friends, but consider the last real conversation you had about your vagina. For many of us, the joking covers up something that we are not able to talk about seriously. The longer we keep joking, the harder it becomes to have a serious conversation. Consider shar-ing the traumas that you may have sustained but cannot talk about because of the silence we maintain around our sexuality. Whether those traumas come from childbirth, forced or painful sexual encoun-ters, or the cultural shame associated with genitalia, the majority of women silently bear the burden of unspoken conversations about their vaginal life.

Educate yourself, trust your freedom, and start looking for ways to have those conversations. Allowing yourself the privilege of under-standing one of the most complex and highly innervated areas of the body is a wonderful way to access the pleasure capacity we are all born with. Giving both voice and names to the vagina and other sexual organs might just be one of the most sexually respectful acts we can commit in our lifetime, and it is sure to awaken our curiosity and capacity for pleasure.

When it comes to pleasure, orgasm is the holy grail. So as we talk about pleasure, let's spend a moment focusing on orgasm. Having all but lost my ability to orgasm in the morass of my horrible sexual exploits in college, I was amazed at how the freedom and curiosity that characterized my affair with Michel brought this innate capacity flooding back to me. All of the stories of French lovers lasting through the night were true, and my orgasmic potential exploded in ways that I would not have believed possible.

Everybody wants to orgasm, yet orgasm is elusive for millions of women. Many studies, including a 2004 global study on sexual behavior that involved 27,000 participants from thirty countries, have revealed that orgasmic dysfunction is the norm rather than the exception.[11] One-third of all women have never experienced an orgasm during intercourse, and a second third rarely experience orgasm.[12] And orgasmic dysfunction is not just a woman's story; similar numbers of men suffer from a range of issues that hinder their ability to experience orgasm.[13]

Orgasm is a natural biological response that is built into our bodies, yet it often gets buried by time and cultural conditioning. The rate of anorgasmic women in America is three times higher than it is in Europe, a finding that is both mysterious and revealing when you consider the very different cultural views of sex and sex education in different countries.[14] For many American women, the lack of education about sexual functioning and the rampant misinformation and negative cultural connotations surrounding sexuality have blocked normal sexual curiosity and exploration.

Each orgasm is as unique as the individual experiencing it. The wide variety of intensities, locations, and stimuli that contribute to orgasm play a big part in the difficulty many women experience identifying what their own orgasm feels like. When my daughter was first becoming sexually active, she came to me one day and said, "I'm not sure, but I think I might have had an orgasm." I asked her to describe what it was like. She went on to explain that there was a sensation of building pressure and then this explosive moment in which the pressure was released. "Yep," I said, "that's it."

Studies have found that the confusion about experiencing orgasm goes both ways: some women claim to have had an orgasm and show no bodily response, while other women who do have classic responses like vaginal contractions and a racing heart believe that nothing has happened.[15] The modern mythology (and pornography) of orgasm looms so large that many women are not even sure how to identify their own.

What makes orgasm so elusive is that it is not under our conscious control. Orgasm cannot be forced. Methods of cajoling seem to backfire. Betty Dodson, the famous sex therapist who used to hold masturbation sessions for women, taught that orgasm is where the body takes over.[16] This makes sense because the experience of orgasm often feels like a burst of pleasure, bliss, and emotional and physical release. In fact, the moment of orgasm creates such a complete release that the brain center that controls anxiety and fear is switched off.[17]

Giving yourself over to orgasm is a leap. Some people describe it as the same feeling you get when you plummet from the top of a roller coaster. Taking the plunge requires the ability to be completely in the present moment and to feel entirely safe. It isn't surprising then that your chances of having an orgasm are much better on your own than with a partner. Part of the difficulty many women have with achieving orgasm—and even recognizing their own pleasure response—is that they are afraid to touch themselves. Many people spend their lives married to people with whom they can't even say the word *masturbate*, let alone imagine sharing the act. Not being able to disclose or trust their sexuality holds their orgasm hostage.

The good news is that the more orgasms you have, the more orgasms you're likely to have in the future. Learning about your own sexual response and developing your orgasmic potential will bring both immediate gratification and long-term satisfaction. As they do for any skill-based human motor function, all bodies come equipped with the tools for orgasm. Yet without the proper education and opportunity to practice, many people never successfully achieve the synergy of mind, body, and spirit that releases this very unique and revelatory experience. It is a quest worthy of our time and attention.

While there are hundreds of scientific studies that demonstrate the physical, mental, and emotional health benefits of orgasmic pleasure, perhaps the strongest, most life-changing reason to pursue an evolving relationship with orgasm is the spiritual connection it opens for us. Indeed, the French term for orgasm, *le petit mort*, which means "small death," describes the process in which we let go of our ego-driven self and experience a divine connection with our partner—a connection in which the universe is revealed.

Studies have confirmed that as many as one in twenty individuals has a transcendent experience in orgasm. The range of experiences cited were unique and included a shift in space and time; a sense of timelessness and vast emptiness; a sense of electric, light-filled bodies; and a transformation of self and other converging in intersecting paths of spirit and sexuality.[18] For many people, the spiritual awakening that comes through transcendent orgasm is life-changing. It reorganizes their beliefs about sexuality and God. There are some historical notions that the forbidden fruit in the Garden of Eden was actually orgasm because it held the secret that connection to the divine is achieved through our natural capacity to connect to each other.

Of all the life experiences that open the doorway to intensely spiritual experiences, sex is the one readily available to ordinary people, even those with no prior experience of spirituality. Orgasm transforms our physical body into a vessel of energy. Our cellular physical boundaries fade as our bodies become vehicles transporting us into experiences that connect us to the universal energy that is our spiritual source.

Finding this transcendent orgasm might be as simple as discovering your innate ability to let go. You can begin by developing a daily routine of learning to physically recognize where and how stress lives in your body and practice releasing it. Not only is this a secret of graceful aging, but also, more profoundly, the practice of release opens us to the mysterious and compelling territory of experiencing sexual pleasure. Releasing our control is simultaneously the path to the transcendent, mysterious human orgasm and the reward.

For many of us, the terrain of our sexuality has been limited to intercourse, and our internal maps for intercourse are often composed of straight lines to what we think the destination should be: orgasm. But when we view intercourse and sexuality this way, we lose out on all there is to experience during the complex, mysterious journey to untapped pleasure.

Giving up the destination and lingering in all that makes up the "outercourse" of our sexual selves offers us a new world to explore. Slowing down while actively engaging in what is happening during sex is often the key to fully mature and fulfilling intercourse. Ask anyone who has ever had their lover's hands slowly linger over each part: the pleasure is in the process.

>> Remember the last great scavenger hunt you enjoyed—how the treasure at the end was all the more enjoyable because of the discoveries along the way. Mapping the curves and valleys of your lover's body with a hand gliding over sweet- or spicy-scented-oiled skin will surprise you. The nape of the neck, the rise of a hip, the indent of the knee—all contain sensations that can unlock your libido in ways you might not expect. Inhaling your partner is an ancient form of kissing. Learning to linger in the outercourse of sexuality will transform your connection to your partner and, perhaps even more deeply, your ability to open to the sexual experience itself.

Working toward developing your pleasure capacity and having the courage to witness your unique yet universal connection to all humanity through your erotic self is the path of mastery in human life. Freeing ourselves from the constraints of our culture and embracing our sexual selves as the wise energetic transformers they are is a path to peace inside and out. We are all born with the birthright to know our divine source through the physical love of the bodies we were born into. This is the fertile ground at the root of healing and the place where love is born.

Mutual pleasure is the energy that powers every love relationship. Think about the sun, the only passive source of energy the earth receives. All the light and all the heat that exist without human effort begin there. The idea of transforming the sun's light into usable energy is at the center of the circle in sustainable thinking. Think of your sexual pleasure as a form of solar energy for your relationship.

Discovering shared pleasure in a relationship is like pouring cement into the foundation. By telling your partner what pleases you and what doesn't, you add vital strength to the foundation. This information is what helps intimacy work. For many couples—in fact, I would say most—intimacy is a completely empty space; there is no information in the container of their relationship on which to draw. So, in a void of understanding, they stumble through what they think should make intimacy work, relying on alcohol, porn, and other distractions to make themselves feel good—all without articulating to themselves or each other what it is they like.

For intimacy to work, both people have to be willing to understand their own pleasure response and stop holding the other person responsible for pressing the right buttons. This then creates space in which each person can explore and add to the container what feels good for them. Otherwise, if we aren't adding to the container, blame and hostility fill the empty space of intimacy. I have noticed a telling coincidence between people who don't orgasm and people who divorce. While sharing pleasure alone is not enough to keep a moribund relationship alive, the inability to move toward it is enough to kill even a healthy relationship.

There are many who hang on to the mythology that good sex is just something that happens to you if the relationship is right or, worse still, if you are "meant for each other." Know that cultivating a life with someone that holds the magic of shared pleasure is a lifework. No other single work in life will repay you so profoundly each and every time you share it. When the container of our relationship is strong, we feel safer exploring the outer limits of pleasure, where experiences of the body can become experiences of the spirit and teach us about our truest selves.

As we become more attuned to pleasure, both our own and our partner's, we begin to rely more on the physical conversation in our relationship. Words may bring us to this place of understanding pleasure, but the times when words don't work, when we can hardly remember why we keep showing up for our relationship, are times begging for the best sex we might ever have. It isn't the easiest sex to initiate: you both have to get past your egos to let the wisdom of your bodies lead.

Here's something I have found to be true: my verbal conversations with my husband have more depth, intimacy, and real listening when we have a physical conversation first. Sex connects two people in a way that words can sometimes confuse. We seriously underrate pleasure as a medium of communication. We dismiss our bodies and their needs as being unequal to, or at least baser than, the thoughts floating around in our heads. But my body is more honest than my mind—*if* I am willing to listen to it. Left to their own devices, the stories in my mind will build castles out of sand and destroy empires.

Have the conversation with your body first. Stop talking about it, and let your body's wisdom lead you into a language of touch. It has the power to communicate what is behind words. A physical, but not necessarily sexual, conversation is the open door to a more emotionally connected relationship. The pleasure that comes from building and strengthening this connection over time is often beyond words.

3

FINDING YOUR NORMAL

During the years I've worked in sexuality education, reassuring people that they are sexually normal has been part of my job. For years on my website I kept an "Ask the Loveologist" column, where I would receive many questions from people wanting to know, essentially, "Am I sexually normal?" In response I would cite the most extensive sexual research that was compiled in the twentieth century, the Kinsey Reports—*Sexual Behavior in the Human Male* (1948) and *Sexual Behavior in the Human Female* (1953)—which demonstrated that sexual normalcy exists on such a broad spectrum, with so many preferences, activities, and experiences, that there's really no one definition of normal. Most people are engaging in all kinds of sexual behaviors.[1]

I believe it's true that there is no "normal" when it comes to sex. Still, after my husband and I have had especially wild sex, I'll sometimes find myself covering my eyes and asking myself, "Who was that?" The woman I am in bed seems so different from the woman I am during everyday life that I almost feel as if I am two different people. Then, even though I know better, I ask myself, "Is this normal?" There's a way in which our intimacy in that charged, erotic space fails us as soon as we leave the bed. After such extreme pleasure, I feel vulnerable and uncomfortable as I try to find the bridge back to mundane life.

I suspect my reaction will seem familiar to many people. Our sexuality is often not very well integrated with the rest of our identity. Who we are when we're at work or with our family may be very different from who we are when we are having passionate sex. There's a good reason for this. We have to take on different roles and behaviors in different situations in order to function in the world. Yet as a consequence, certain roles become more familiar or habitual than others, and after years of being an employee, a wife or a husband, a mother or a father, we often find it hard to relate to the other, wilder parts of ourselves. Even though our sexuality is fundamentally integral to who we are, it is not unusual to become so distanced from it that it no longer seems normal. This wondering about our normality is itself totally normal when it comes to fully embodying our erotic soul. Sadly, though, we often get hung up on the question, and as a result, our health and relationships suffer, and sex stops working.

In the previous chapter, we saw how reawakening our pleasure sense can guide us to explore our erotic souls. That may lead us into unexpected new territories, which can be rich with potential for healing and growth. Yet one intense encounter that leads us too far outside our comfort zone, sometimes even a fantasy, can take our sexuality, in our own eyes, outside the bounds of "normal" and into perversion. Alternatively, we might feel perfectly normal ourselves but hear other people tell us that we are not. And if we are in a relationship with someone very different from us, we might start to wonder, "Is there something wrong with my partner? Is there something wrong with me? We're so different. How can we both be normal?"

In this chapter, I'll offer a simple model to help facilitate new thinking about sexual identity and move you beyond the question of what is normal. A couple of key ideas that may help clarify include *community* and *context*: without a *community* in which we can be open and honest about sex, we lose *context* for our sexual feelings and behaviors, which can make us wonder about every sexual experience. Moreover, isolation from one another and from our own sexual selves often leads to sexual dysfunction, which may make us feel that it isn't just our behaviors or fantasies but also our bodies themselves that are not normal. Unfortunately, there are people in the medical and pharmaceutical industries who make money by encouraging us to think just that.

I'll also discuss the forms dysfunction takes in both men and women (surprise: they are not so different) and will map out a route for moving beyond a model of disease and dysfunction toward an ability to feel more and to open to intense erotic pleasure. Shifting the line of questioning about our erotic selves from "What is normal?" toward "What is functional? And what works for me?" is a worthy goal.

The word *normal* suggests the middle of the road, the median or average. It might even lean toward something that is predictable, if not a little bit boring. But compelling, passionate sex is not predictable or boring and by definition exceeds our expectations. After any intense sexual experiences, whether pleasurable or not, we often feel, "This can't be normal"—and in a way, we are right. Exceptional experiences live outside the lines of our daily lives; they are more abnormal than normal. Especially when it comes to our erotic life, we often lack both the context and the communication skills to process and digest the range of extraordinary experiences that make sex great.

In the previous chapter, I mentioned the affair I had in my twenties with the Frenchman, Michel, who showed me the extreme of how *good* sex can feel. I learned a great deal from him about my erotic capacity. I learned that I could maintain my desire, even all night, that there was such a thing as multiple orgasms, and that I could have them. I learned how sexual pleasure can share a border with pain and how to lean toward the pleasure side of that border. I learned new positions and new ways of touching my body and my partner's. And when it was all over, I found myself wondering about the wide range of pleasure I had experienced, which was so far removed from my earlier sexual experiences that the question came to me, "Is this normal?"

More frequently I have asked that question when sex isn't working—when neither my husband nor I have the desire, or when only one of us does, or when we're too tired, angry, or distracted to be intimate with each other. The question about normal came up in a big way after I started having kids and the changes in my body put an end to some of its natural capacities, like lubrication and even libido. I wondered then, too, "Is this normal?"

In both cases, the issue of normality came up when I had stepped outside of the context of my previously known sexual self—when I simply did not have knowledge or experience to help me make sense of what I was going through. Lacking context in our erotic journey generates our doubts about normality. Generally, our fears about not being normal are signs of erotic maturation, the natural growing pains that come from creating a wider personal range of what normal can mean. But when I was in the midst of this questioning—and I think this is true for all of us—I suffered sexual doubts and, worse still, felt isolated and alone with them.

Over the years, as I've helped thousands of people with the widest variety of sexual issues, I've discovered some of the context that I was missing. In particular, there are two personality attributes that help provide some clarity and context for understanding our own sexual identities and how they impact our primary relationships. These attributes live on a continuum and reflect the totality of what exists in the wildly varied field of our human sexuality. The first is how *relational* we are, and the second is how *inhibited* we are.

By *relational*, I mean socially outgoing—comfortable establishing and maintaining relationships and feeling open and connected to people. Highly relational people are all about communicating and relating with others. If you usually enjoy being with other people, talking or sharing experiences or just being together, you are probably more relational. Less relational people may be introverts and, at the more extreme end, hermits. If you usually feel like being by yourself or being quiet, and especially if being with other people feels like work to you, then you are probably less relational.

By *inhibited*, I mean how we might suppress sexual feelings and restrain ourselves from physical contact. Highly inhibited people are not comfortable with physical contact of any kind, especially sexual, while highly uninhibited people enjoy pushing comfort boundaries and experimenting sexually.

Before we go on, it's important to address the role cultural relativity plays in the terms we're using. How relational or inhibited we see ourselves as is always compared to the norms of the culture we live in.

At different times and in different places, being inhibited might reflect very different kinds of behavior. For example, a woman in Victorian England who wore restrictive corsets and did not allow herself to be touched might have considered her sexuality to be totally normal, but if someone did the same thing today, we would call her highly inhibited. Similarly, a woman living in Egypt today might place herself on the uninhibited side because she sometimes does not cover all of her hair when she's out in public. Even within your own culture, existence at the margins might seem odd to the majority but still be healthy and right for you.

These two characteristics, inhibition and relationality, can work together in some ways, but they are not the same thing. I find it helpful to think of them as two axes on a grid. Let's call it the Sexual Identity Grid. The horizontal axis of this grid is a self-reported measurement of one's comfort with their sexuality: on the far left end are people who are totally sexually inhibited, and on the far right are those who perceive themselves as sexually uninhibited or experimental. The vertical axis is a measurement of how emotionally relational we are: at the top of the axis are people for whom relationships are all consuming, and at the bottom are those who self-identify as not relationally connected.

THE SEXUAL IDENTITY GRID

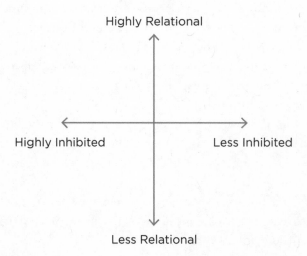

When I put inhibition and relationality together on the grid like this, four sexual personality types emerge that reflect core aspects of a person's sexual experience and identity. In the upper right is someone who is both highly relational and highly uninhibited. This is a person who is at ease in their body, at ease with other people, a person who likes to spend time with someone else, touching and being touched. If you've seen the 2004 movie *Kinsey*, you know an example of this type: Alfred Kinsey, as portrayed in that movie, belongs in this area. The film also showed the danger of this personality type: Kinsey was hyper-relational and hypersexual, so that he actually ended up damaging his intimate relationships.

In the lower right of the grid is someone who is uninhibited but not relational. This person likes to spend time alone, but when they are with a partner, they are interested in exploring their sexuality and experimenting with sensation. In more extreme cases, this could be somebody who enjoys looking for casual hookups online, perhaps experimenting with BDSM (bondage, domination, sadomasochism) or other fetishes. This might also be the more familiar figure of the disengaged spouse who isn't getting what they want sexually out of the marriage and turns to pornography or extramarital affairs to fill the gap.

People who are sexually inhibited and highly relational belong in the upper left. These are social people who love to be in groups but don't want to be touched. I seem to find a lot of them in volunteer groups or social and political activist groups. If you've been active in that kind of group, have you noticed the truly kind and open people who want to help everyone with everything but shy away when you get too personal with them?

Finally, in the lower left are people who are both inhibited and nonrelational. They like to be alone, and they're not that excited about sex. This might seem like a gloomy part of the grid to be in, but many of these people simply enjoy their own thoughts and company and prize the space and freedom they get by not giving too much energy to relationships. Many of our greatest thinkers probably belong in this zone.

None of these personality types is better than the others; they each have strengths and weaknesses. And although locating yourself on the grid can be helpful in providing a larger context for your sexual identity, it can also lead back to the same old questions—Is it normal to be in this part of the grid?—which is not helpful. It is most useful to use the grid to ask different questions, not just about where you find yourself but also about where you are *in relation* to your partner and the other important people in your life. The real value of the Sexual Identity Grid is in helping you visualize relationships.

I first conceived this grid when I needed help understanding my own relationship. I've always lived in the highly relational and more uninhibited part of the grid, and after my affair with Michel, who was even more uninhibited, I was pulled further in that direction. My husband, on the other hand, has always been more comfortable on the opposite side of the grid—both more inhibited and less relational. The biggest challenge in our marriage had always been bridging that distance—and not only in our sexual life. There were many ways that these differences kept us apart, and in the early days, when we focused only on the differences, it seemed impossible to find a meeting place and to preserve our commitment. During the time I was with Michel, my husband and I were separated. We didn't know what would happen next or whether it was worth trying to save our marriage. And it didn't help when he learned about my affair and how excited I'd been by someone closer to my own relational and uninhibited "normal."

My husband was wounded, and his trust in me was shattered. Things did not look good for us.

During the years of therapy that followed, I began to approach our differences in a new way. For one thing, those very differences and our courage to not become like each other have consistently provided a mighty fuel for our passion. Working to understand more about *how* we were different and the nature of the distance between us opened the door to a path that would allow us to reach each other. Over time, that thinking led me to the Sexual Identity Grid and helped us learn more about what we have to do to keep loving each other. We solved the problem of finding each other in different areas of this grid as we each moved closer to the center, where the distance between our preferences could be bridged.

The center is a place of balance and healing in many spiritual traditions. Think of the Middle Way in Buddhism or the importance of alignment in yoga. There is nothing wrong with being in whatever corner of the grid you're comfortable in, but the grid is most useful as a map to help you reach the other people in your life. And to do that, you will often need to move toward the common ground at the center.

So try this: first, locate yourself on the grid. Don't overthink it or spend too much time on it. Just put an X where your intuition says you belong. Then put four more Xs on the grid for people you're close to, including your spouse or partner if you have one. Try to answer the following questions as you do so:

- How comfortable are you in the neighborhood on the grid where you've located yourself? Do you feel like part of a community here? Do you feel excluded?

- How does your location on the grid help you to explore your sexuality? How does it keep you safe?

- How close are you to the center of the grid? How does that distance shape your experience of your sexuality?

- If you placed someone you love in a different area of the grid, consider how you relate to that person. Is it easy for you? Difficult? What strategies do you use?

- Notice the length of the line connecting you to your spouse or partner (or to someone else you're very close to). What energy does this distance bring to your relationship? In what ways is this energy generative? In what ways is it draining?

The Sexual Identity Grid is my context for thinking about how people relate to each other sexually. It is really the lack of this context that complicates the question of what is normal for so many of us. It doesn't help that our formal sexual education is limited and that there is very little authentic discussion about our sexual behaviors. That is to say, we don't know what is normal for other people because we don't generally experience our sexuality in community.

This is least true for those whose sexual lives are outside of the typical heterosexual model. In the context of lesbian, gay, bisexual, or transgender identities, or BDSM preferences, the clear intention of people who live in these more marginalized groups allows them to relate more deeply and frequently through their sexual identity. In important ways, many people who identify themselves through more marginalized gender or sexual identities tend to be more comfortable living through their sexual identity day to day. In other words, their everyday identities are more seamlessly integrated with their erotic selves, making it easier to move from intense erotic experiences back to everyday life without having to stop to wonder, "Who was that?"

The secrecy and shame around our erotic selves is why this question of what is normal keeps haunting us. The less isolated we are—the more information we have, the more willing we are to go out and find new resources and learn about the real universe of sexual behavior—the more likely we are to keep following our pleasure and have sex that isn't stymied by worries over what is normal and what isn't. Sex that works depends on our being able to trust ourselves, and our ability to trust ourselves depends on understanding who we are and how we relate to the people around us. Once we understand that, we stop asking, "Is this normal?" and start asking, "Is this working for me? Is it working for my relationship? Would it work better if I changed?"

Unfortunately, in our culture, many people are quick to go looking for prescriptions and quick fixes when they notice something unusual about themselves. The United States is one of two countries (the other is New Zealand) in the world that allows pharmaceutical companies to advertise directly to consumers. This fact might well explain why our total population, which represents only 5 percent of the world's population, consumes 75 percent of all the pharmaceutical drugs sold globally.[2] It also explains how more and more everyday human experiences are being seen as "treatable" health conditions. Turning ordinary life experiences into treatable conditions has impacted everything from shyness to restless legs. Without a doubt, there are conditions for which medical attention is absolutely necessary, and potential symptoms should always be discussed with a doctor. However, there are many ways in which the pathologization of our bodies, especially their erotic functions, can hinder rather than help our healing.

An excellent example of this phenomenon is what's now being called female sexual dysfunction (FSD). Many women—most clinical studies cite the statistic of 43 percent—will at some point in their lives be affected by a range of FSD symptoms that include vaginal dryness, pain with intimacy, and loss of libido. It is difficult to decipher which symptoms beget which others, and it is even harder to unravel the emotional, mental, and spiritual impacts of this extremely common, yet rarely discussed, condition.

The medical research that resulted in the rise of Viagra in the 1990s was partly responsible for the impetus to identify and name this "parallel female syndrome" to male sexual dysfunction. A 2014 study collected data on thousands of women's self-reported frequency of a group of common symptoms that are the hallmarks of FSD; it was this first study that generated the statistic that 43 percent of women had sexual dysfunction.[3] That number was later refuted by the authors, but this study was the seed that firmly planted the idea that dysfunctional female sexuality can be diagnosed as an illness, with its own medical code.

This idea is the foundation on which the multibillion-dollar industry of sexual dysfunction has been built in the last twenty years. Inspired by the billions of dollars of income that Viagra and similar drugs have generated in the male sexual dysfunction arena, pharmaceutical companies have lobbied for the implementation of diagnostic or medical codes that pathologize female sexuality as well. As I write this, Sprout Pharmaceuticals has just received U.S. Food and Drug Administration (FDA) approval to release its drug flibanserin, an antidepressant that had previously been rejected by the FDA three times, as a treatment for FSD.[4] Only two days after the approval, Sprout, a company of less than forty employees, was sold for $1 billion, easily surpassing a $100 million initial investment spent mostly on an elaborate social media campaign equating a dubious drug's approval to equal rights for women.[5]

Meanwhile millions of women have been won over to the pathology mentality. The personal and private exploration of the erotic self has become instead for many women an expensive and often risky ordeal of experimental medical treatments that leave them feeling hopeless and used. From the Orgasmatron, a device that promised control over orgasm through the use of an electrical probe inserted directly into the spinal column, to a popular new form of female genital plastic surgery, women have become willing to try almost anything in the name of a "cure."

Some women believe that all of the media hype surrounding flibanserin both exaggerates the prevalence of FSD and creates additional anxiety among women, making them believe they need treatment for their sexuality or lack of it. "The messages are aimed at medicalizing normal conditions and also preying on the insecurity of both the clinician and the patient," says Dr. Fugh Berman of Georgetown University.[6]

Many more physicians and researchers doubt whether these conditions are treatable with drugs, even if they really are medical conditions. Leonore Tiefer, PhD, a sex therapist in New York, incensed by the medicalization of female sexuality, has started an advocacy and lobbying group called the New View Campaign. The group's argument is that normal sexual functioning cannot be reduced to the physiological treatment of individual body parts. Female sexual functioning can only be understood and healed within the context of the relationship and society in which it occurs. The quality of communication and the safety that arise out of sustained healthy connection are as essential for many women as the right balance of hormones.

Even if a pill is truly effective at raising levels of desire for women, the question of the vitality of the relationship will continue to impact our access to and enjoyment of physical intimacy. The old saying that men need sex to feel connected and women need connection to feel sexual provides a good hint at an actual solution to increasing female libido. Dismissing the critical social, political, and economic conditions that define a woman's life under the umbrella term "psychogenic causes" ignores the profound and perhaps deepest reality of a woman's sexuality.

The one good thing that has come out of the flibanserin debacle is that now we might have an opportunity to have real conversations about female libido, a conversation that can lead to real solutions that have nothing to do with drugs. Why don't we begin with some basic sex education and dispel a few persistent myths about how libido works, as well as how it changes?

The persistent and harmful belief that sexual desire is or should be spontaneous is where the trouble starts. We all remember those initial early stirrings of sexual hunger—when just being near our crush of the month unleashed an animal inside of us or when the biologically driven stage of falling in love triggered the frenzied, rip-the-clothes-off feelings. Who doesn't love that kind of spontaneous eruption of desire? It's like surfing a giant wave or dancing around a bonfire. So yes, there are times, rare and beautiful as they are, when our libido spontaneously takes us on a fantastic ride, sometimes resulting in an over-the-top orgasm.

And then there is life, with jobs and careers, bills, health and fitness goals, pets, children, and in-laws. Somehow spontaneous sexual desire doesn't always find its way onto this list. This is why we have to start working toward a new and more reliable form of libido. As adults, we have to both want and learn to generate our capacity for desire.

But this is where the libido story falls apart for most women. A participant in the flibanserin trials said, "Once I started, it wasn't an issue. It was getting me started." Another participant said, "I hate having to 'wind myself up' to do it. It makes me feel broken."[7] These comments reflect the real problem with female libido: most women don't understand that what makes desire work over the long term is being willing to own and cultivate our erotic souls.

It is a big leap to take responsibility for our own erotic impulses. It is much easier to let them lie dormant under a giant stack of old guilt or sexual wounds, emotional disconnection from our partner, silent shame about our body image, or just having no idea how to access a fantasy life. Cultivating our erotic soul is grown-up business that requires both curiosity and commitment, and many women equate the difficulty of that work with being broken. We know now that desire is not usually the leader, as waking up our capacity to be aroused is enough to ignite desire. And arousal is available through any of our senses if we go looking for it.

Giving up the longing for spontaneous desire to take hold of you and moving instead toward *cultivating* responsive desire is the only pill you need to take. Not only will you avoid the pain and embarrassment of frequent fainting spells (a side effect of flibanserin that will not help your libido), you will also forge exciting new pathways in your brain and actually get to the passion we all truly want.

Isolation can magnify our concerns about what is normal, making it seem as though we alone have this huge, insoluble problem to deal with. When it comes to sex, this effect can be especially pernicious since there is often such shame about discussing anything sexual. Sexual dysfunction flourishes in these conditions of silence and shame. When I was writing my "Ask a Loveologist" column, I got to be the one people reached out to with concerns they felt they couldn't share with anyone else. It allowed me to see that we are all worried about essentially the same things when it comes to our bodies and their sexual functions. If you have some concern about your body, the truth is probably this: not only is that thing you are concerned about normal, your worry about it is normal too.

Sexual worries are surprisingly consistent even across gender boundaries. Consider the topics I received questions about most frequently:

Women	Men
No desire	No desire
Concerns about vagina appearance	Concerns about penis size
Vaginal atrophy	Difficulty maintaining an erection
Vaginal dryness	Premature ejaculation
Pain (pelvic, vaginal)	

My readers' questions did a lot to inform my idea of what "normal" means. As you read a few sample letters, along with my responses, I believe you'll see as well that what is normal is really a much bigger field than we tend to think.

For example, I received many letters from women concerned about their inability to orgasm. Here is one that could stand in for hundreds, followed by my response:

Q *I am a twenty-one-year-old female. I can't seem to come when I have sex, and that bothers my partner because he doesn't think he's done his part. I mean, it's great sex, but I just can't come. What's wrong with me?*

A Thanks for this question. There is nothing wrong with you. This is a concern that affects about a third of all women. Of the women who do have orgasms, many of them only orgasm occasionally and without really understanding why it happens or doesn't. Opening up to the experience of orgasm is a process, and having a partner who is interested in and supportive of your process is a gift.

It is much more common for women to be able to orgasm by themselves than in their partnerships. Many couples struggle with this reality and long for a solution to sharing intimacy and pleasure. Experiencing orgasm with another person requires trust—both in yourself and in your partner. Sharing deep sexual pleasure equally requires deeply letting go and vulnerability. It is essential that your relationship feel safe. Orgasm is an experience that you can't force, so a good place to start is by letting go of worry and feeling all the sensations that happen during your sexual experience.

Understanding a bit about how the brain functions when it comes to orgasm might shed some light on what happens when the arousal process turns off during your intimate times. One important study of the brain's process during orgasm shows that when a woman reaches orgasm, something unexpected happens: much of her brain goes silent. Brain regions responsible for everything from her sense of self-control to her moral reasoning and judgment all get turned down in the moments of intense arousal.[8]

"Fear and anxiety need to be avoided at all costs if a woman wishes to have an orgasm; we knew that, but now we can see it happening in the depths of the brain," said researcher Gert Holstege at the 2005 meeting of the European Society for Human Reproduction and Development. "At the moment of orgasm, women do not have any emotional feelings."[9]

While some brain areas get shut down, others are activated. The production of oxytocin, the love and bonding hormone, jumps fourfold at orgasm. The researchers also found heightened activity in the critical part of the brain's reward circuitry that may mediate orgasmic pleasure in women.[10] Such activity may connect a female's sexual pleasure with the emotional bond she feels with her partner.

Getting your brain to release you for this remarkable experience is more an activity of surrender than it is a push. As you have seen from your own experience, trying only makes it less available. Use your boyfriend's interest to your advantage; rather than making your time together center on the orgasm, spend it exploring what feels good. Oral sex is one of the first doorways for many women to experience orgasm with a partner. Even mutual hand stimulation can open your eyes to what feels really good.

Like most things, when you take your eye off the goal and get really involved in the process, you start enjoying the journey. And enjoyment—not reaching some preconceived idea of how things should be—is what it's all about.

I also received many letters from women and men who were concerned because their libido did not match their partner's. Having a different level of sex drive than your partner's doesn't mean there's anything wrong with you. Not all sex drives are created equal—that's normal—and our relationship to our sexuality is heavily influenced by our gender, age, and overall health. For many men, the signals to their sex drive are hanging in their pants. Their body speaks directly. For women, though, sexual desire is often more subtle and complex. If your sex drive is different from your partner's, that doesn't mean there's anything wrong with you. Rethinking your approach to desire is perhaps the most productive way of cultivating a stronger libido, if you decide that is what you want.

For me, desire is usually a product of my decision to go looking for it. While I do remember times, mostly in the middle of my fertility cycle, when it was just there, unbidden like hunger, more often than not, I have to trust that by opening up to the places where arousal is sparked, I will feel my way to the place within me that desires and, on a good day, even lusts. By reversing the idea that desire precedes and ignites arousal and instead letting arousal trigger desire, we begin to unlock the mystery of where body and mind meet.

Recognizing that desire can be ignited through the process of receptivity encourages both partners to foster emotional connection. The dance is in creating and emphasizing the places where our desire multiplies, igniting more desire. Oftentimes, however, our bodies do not respond reliably despite our desire. Dryness and pain for women and erectile dysfunction for men are common concerns.

Here is one representative letter, followed by my response.

Q *I have been having pain on my vagina for a long time and have tried all the over-the-counter medicines I could find. Nothing is helping, and it hurts just to pee and wipe myself. Sometimes the burning is bad when I just sit for too long or wear jeans. I can't even think about being sexual. I don't know what to do.*

A What you are describing sounds painfully familiar to many women who, like you, often go without a diagnosis or treatment. Vaginal pain is a fairly common condition. In a recent study, 30 percent of women reported pain during vaginal sex; this finding suggests that pain in the vaginal area impacts over 40 million women in the United States alone.[11] Although there are still some physicians who are unfamiliar with this condition and its treatments, awareness and the range of treatment options are growing. If you have chronic or recurring genital pain, you should find a physician who can help you and rule out easily treatable causes.

Chronic pain on the outside of the vaginal opening, which is the vulvar region, is called *vulvodynia*. Symptoms include the burning mentioned, plus itching, stinging, rawness, soreness, and painful intercourse. Women who have struggled with recurring bacterial or yeast infections have a higher risk of vulvodynia, as do those who have a history of sexual abuse. However, most women with vulvodynia have no known factors that are associated with the condition.

A similar condition, called *vulvar vestibulitis*, may cause pain only when pressure is applied to the area surrounding the vulva. Another related condition, *vaginismus*, might also be considered if the muscles around and in the vagina tend to spasm. It is not an easy call, as vaginal pain can cause spasms and spasms can cause pain.

For many women, the first symptoms of these conditions come with their first experiences of intercourse, which is one of the reasons many women don't talk about it or seek help.

Sometimes basic changes like switching to cotton underwear and giving up tight-fitting clothes can make a difference. Avoiding petrochemical irritants in douches, soaps, detergents, and lubricants can also make a big difference for some women. Others have success with the use of topical creams and hormones. Still others, especially those with high urine oxalate levels, have reported eliminating pain through a low-oxalate diet. Many women have also found relief through biofeedback programs, physical therapy, and relaxation programs.

Education is a good friend when it comes to conditions that impact our daily lives. In the case of vaginal pain, there are excellent website resources and books to help you better understand what is happening in your body and take the steps to deal with it effectively. The National Vulvodynia Association maintains an exhaustive site that offers resources, medical referrals, and online education.

The best advice I can give any woman who is struggling with pain is not to be afraid and not to just accept it. Pain can make us feel helpless and even isolated, because our pain is something we experience alone. But everybody experiences pain sooner or later. Do the research and find the support you need to move toward solutions. We are always our own best advocates.

Lack of lubrication is another concern I received many letters about:

Q *For the past month or so, every time my husband and I have sex, I can't come. What is wrong with me? There's always a lack of natural lubrication. We also have a three-month-old baby.*

A As a sexuality educator, I get lots of questions about vaginal lubrication. Many women and their partners find vaginal lubrication rather enigmatic—and for good reason. Most textbook explanations of the "mechanics of sex" don't mention it. Polite conversations steer clear of it. And frankly, lubrication as a symbol of desire and readiness for lovemaking is quite subtle; for example, it isn't quite as obvious as its male counterpart, an erection. But don't let the subtlety of lubrication fool you. It plays a huge role in how women experience feelings of arousal and the physical sensations of lovemaking.

Without lubrication, women can feel as if their desire must be low, or the sensation of touch can be irritating or even painful. You mention that you are a new mother. Lack of lubrication is a normal experience for new mothers. For many women, the same hormones that help promote a healthy pregnancy and breast milk production also cause a lack of vaginal lubrication. This is natural and not a cause for alarm. And it doesn't require that women cease being intimate with their partners during and after a pregnancy. Throughout history women have used a variety of lubricants to help them ease into enjoying intimacy.

Keep in mind that oftentimes the physiological state of "not getting wet" is accompanied by a lack of sexual drive; our natural lubrication also signals that we are aroused. These body memories are stored deep in our psyche. Even the best lubricant in the world cannot adequately do its job if you are not ready to be penetrated or if your only associations with the act are fearful and painful.

One of my clients shared with me the unfortunate story of her husband's poorly executed penile implant, which left him both significantly shorter and with reduced erectile function. She wrote that she and her husband "have been unable to shake the anger and hopelessness, and this issue has ruined our lives."

As I thought about the gravity of her experience, I remembered one time early in my sex education career when one of the women attending my workshop shared a similar story. After a complicated hysterectomy, she had been unable to have the same kind of orgasm that she had regularly enjoyed throughout her life. I remember her despair also described in terms of "ruining my life."

Indeed, the association between sexual incapacity and ruin is painfully common. The late husband of an old friend of mine chose to not treat prostate cancer, which ended up killing him, for fear of the sexual incapacity he might experience as a side effect of treatment. Having worked with both cancer patients and survivors, I can say that his fear was not unfounded. Cancer and its treatments join many other illnesses and treatments that wreak havoc on our sexual desire, libido, and capacity for pleasure. And while physical ailments might have a more obvious effect on our sex lives, we are stymied even more often by all varieties of emotional estrangement and disappointed expectations that prevent us from exposing our most intimate vulnerability and exploring our capacity for pleasure.

There are some who believe that the cure to this situation lies in questioning our expectations of how often we can rightly look forward to having great sex. Maybe a handful of profoundly erotic exchanges should be a fair limit for our sexual ambitions in a lifetime, they say. Others encourage taking up sex education like training for a sport: learning the correct poses, taking the right supplements, studying the latest science, and purchasing the right accessories are all commonly suggested fixes for the sexual ailments of our time.

There is probably some truth to be found in both schools of thought, and yet for too many of us, healing our sexuality remains elusive. We struggle to choose among the plethora of options and wait halfheartedly for some miraculous result that usually doesn't materialize.

Culturally, we are trained to look outward for "solutions" to our "problems," so we often forget about our own ability to transform our experience. Although our bodies do sometimes need the help of a doctor, the labeling that happens around disease need not define who we are and what we are capable of. Instead, we can give more attention to what *we* do—how we think about ourselves and how we use our bodies to relate to each other.

All too often we take for granted the moments of sensual beauty within our daily experiences. Consider these small moments of sensual pleasure that some of the cancer patients I work with listed when we started looking at how their attention to beauty and the senses could forge a path to sexuality:

- stepping into the steam of a hot shower

- soaking in the scented water of a hot bath

- slipping into freshly cleaned sheets

- following your nose to the open door of the bakery

- rubbing your hand down the back of a loved one wearing a soft sweater

- smelling the intoxicating scent of a flower

- tasting warm toast and peanut butter

- catching the scent of hot chocolate or hot coffee before it hits your lips

These daily sensory experiences, which we rarely stop to notice, are stepping-stones to an erotic life that most of us don't ever realize. Once we recognize that we miss much of the flavor and visceral enjoyment life perpetually offers us, we can start to examine how we prevent ourselves from experiencing the sensual pleasure that is available to us regardless of physical disability or emotional discomfort.

I keep coming back to the woman at my workshop years ago whose life was "ruined" because she couldn't orgasm the way she always had. I told her that as long as she kept focusing on what she knew before, there was little room left for her to discover what she didn't yet know about her sexual response.

To the degree that we settle into loss and grief as a lifestyle, we eliminate the curiosity and wonder that can evolve our present situation into one of pleasure. We have to be able to let go of what was in order to be present to the possibility of the life that *is*, in this moment. This is the most profound key to healing sex: that the present moment is where we create the interior space to discover what pleasure is here, now. We are afraid that if we let go of how it was, nothing erotic will be left to replace it. Not so. Believe this: as long as you are living in a human body, it will seek, experience, and evolve pleasure—if you let it. Your body wants you to live in pleasure and is just waiting for your expectations to match your capacity to feel.

Our need to understand and question our sexuality is a double-edged sword. To the degree that it leads us deeper into our erotic selves and closer to our partners, it is an indispensable guide to sexual maturity. But we can also easily get trapped in questions about human sexuality—both our own and others'—so that it becomes debilitating.

This balance point lies on a very thin edge, partly because our sexuality is so little understood or explored. Thus our erotophobia, our personal fear of our own eroticism, arises. The degree to which we distrust or even completely repress our own sexual urges is the degree to which we mistrust the unspoken and potentially dangerous sexuality of others.

This mistrust of our sexual nature has grown to epic proportions in our current cultural view of sexuality. The need to "protect" the family, the church, and the community from the sexual side of human nature has only served to further estrange us from it. This fear even creeps into public policy: there are still six states where it is against the law to sell sex toys, but not guns.

The solution is not the current practice of policing everyone's private sexuality and making our sex lives the subjects of public policy. Rather, it is reinventing the questions that help us understand and live with our sexuality peaceably, which is what the Sexual Identity Grid attempts to do. Those nights when my fantasy life seems to lead me astray, I try to focus on the pleasure that those questions allow me to experience and not get too lost in how I got there. It is a way of trusting myself and abandoning myself to the wilder side of human sexuality that lives in all of us.

>> The places where we are most insecure about our normalcy are also often the same places where we have the least information. By owning and writing down your deepest fear of how you might not be sexually normal, you give yourself a chance to see your fear and, more importantly, own the inquiry as an essential part of your erotic journey. Most people find that their "problems," such as how much or how little they want sex, the fetishes or obsessions that turn them on, or even the ways they can't get aroused, are shared by many. Knowing that your sexual "issues" do not make you unique but rather part of a community of people with the same "issues" can alleviate shame and move you along the road to finding workarounds to whatever is holding you back.

Try it now. Write down what you fear separates you from so-called normal people. If your response feels alarming to you, do some research to find out how many other people share your concerns. Once you realize you are far from alone, new ways of thinking about and working with your sexual issues will emerge.

4

COURAGE

Opening and staying open to a sexual life that works is nothing if not an act of deep courage. While I have been making love to the same man for some thirty years and can honestly say that it has gotten amazingly, increasingly better over the decades, it is important to note that the continuous ecstatic evolution in our sex life exists in direct proportion to the willingness we have both brought to the work of growing up sexually. Like any growing-up journey, you never arrive but are always on the road, which means that you have to be continuously willing to bare more of yourself. You have to be willing to come back to the vulnerability of knowing and exposing your erotic soul, which takes true courage.

It took me a long time to find that courage in my own marriage, and until I found it, to be honest, our sex life held more frustration than it did passion. My erotic potential had awakened in my affair with Michel in my twenties, but it was years until I was able to understand how I could blend the little I knew of my sexual desires with my husband's fledgling approach to his own sexual needs. For years, we were each stuck in our own corners without much language to reach each other. This was long before I had articulated the parameters of the Sexual Identity Grid to help me find a way to meet him in the center. Mostly our early sexual life was a story of longing for the romantic and sexual combustion that we knew was possible, but that continually eluded us. I wanted a sex life that would not only fill me up, as I had experienced with Michel, but that would also unite me with my husband. Yet neither of us had any real skills to create that space, which made much of our sexuality an exercise in approach-avoidance. Most especially, it generated an endless game of scorekeeping, with the points based on who initiated and who rejected.

One thing that I learned in this game is that there is no winner. Although I did more of the initiating early on and he did more of the rejecting, we both shared equally the feeling of shame that happens in a relationship defined by sexual rejection and longing. The defenses we both developed toward each other effectively eliminated our ability to be open with each other—not just sexually but in most every-thing—and our sex life became a minefield where hurt feelings would readily explode. We were stuck in a loop of fear, blame, and rejection.

There was a pivotal moment fifteen years into our marriage, when I was thirty-seven and had all but given up on ever having good sex again. I regularly talked myself into believing that I could maintain a decent marriage and keep my family intact without a satisfying sex life, and I pushed the memories of that early affair out of my head whenever they came back, glaring at my half-truths. Thinking back on that moment now, I recognize it as the one that saved not just my own sexuality but also our marriage. It was the moment we began a shared commitment and journey to grow up sexually. It began with a couple of courageous choices for both of us.

First, my husband came home one day with a Victoria's Secret gift box. This was the first time in all the years we had been together that he'd ever bought lingerie for me. When he offered me that box, I was both stunned and curious. For years, sex, when it happened at all for us, had been a strained and mostly unsatisfying endeavor. I knew that by choosing to accept his gift, which was a real offering to reignite the long-ago burned-out fire between us, I would be saying yes to the possibility of good sex—and to the work of letting go of all the resentment we held for each other around sex. Even though I felt that I had grounds to turn my back—my ego was deeply wounded after years of his rejection—I also knew that if I did, I could be closing the door to what might be the last chance to improve things between us. I knew that how I responded to this gift would be either a new beginning or the end.

I met his courage with my own. I accepted his gift and let go of all of the painful scorekeeping and resentment that our sex life had become. The mutually courageous leap back into a sex life that we both embraced brought with it a surprising new feeling of self-permission and the opportunity to fully embody a sexual self I had abandoned so long ago. Although I couldn't know whether the wild passion I had once experienced would resurface or where our sexual reunion might lead us, I knew for sure that healing our sexual connection would give us the chance to repair what was broken between us, and that made it worthwhile for me to stay in our marriage.

My saying yes and his courage to risk my saying no sparked an amazing sexual affair between us, one that lasted weeks and was unlike anything we'd ever had in our marriage before. Here we were, four kids later, finally discovering an insatiable hunger for each other that had us laying down blankets in front of the fireplace after the kids had gone to bed, staying up until all hours of the night making love in ways we had never tried before. We would call each other during the day and make plans for later that night. I felt out of control and giddy, crossing this bridge to him that I didn't even know existed. Our affair didn't end until I developed honeymoon cystitis—fifteen years after our honeymoon!

What was most miraculous about this time was how the grace of forgiveness enveloped us. With the courage to dive into this deep sexual intimacy, all the years that we had spent in rejection and resentment, keeping score of the searing pain of initiating and being rejected, faded from view. The abandonment and frustration that had for so long defined my experience of marriage increasingly became a distant memory. Forgiveness that is complete changes us so completely that it makes the injuries that define us feel like events that had happened to someone else.

Gradually, our early carnal lust transitioned into a serious dedication to making regular time to be erotic together. Our commitment to develop an enduring intimate life also fueled my own curiosity and willingness to really, finally, grow up sexually—to heal old wounds; take responsibility for my own desire, attitudes, and actions; and learn how to find the passion I once knew, both for my husband's pleasure and my own.

As we began to grow up together sexually, we stopped holding each other hostage, stopped always expecting the other one to be responsible for bringing the sexual desire to the relationship. I stopped waiting for him to say or do the "right things" to make me feel sexy and became adept at finding the sexy place in myself. I also abandoned a persistent idea I had long held: that I could only want sex when the conditions were perfect or when I had the prerequisite feelings of emotional closeness. I began to understand how engaging in physical intimacy actually generated the response I wanted. Letting go of our old assumptions allowed us to meet in the mystery of what might happen when we came together, and it got more exciting and surprising every time.

The freedom of letting go of how I thought it had to be allowed me the space to explore all the things I didn't know about my own sexuality. As I discovered the erotic spaces that sang for me and what kinds of touch lit me up, I was learning a language that let me share how I wanted to be loved. This inspired the same in my husband. After fifteen years, we finally were discovering the ecstatic freedom to be ourselves sexually.

A surprising aspect of this freedom was how it gave me the courage to get over the shame of touching myself in front of him. As we explored the language of saying what we liked and asking for what we wanted, a new sense of possibility was breathed into the narrow routine of sexual behaviors we had for so long limited ourselves to. Even though we had been relying on sexual positions and practices that had always worked, our inability to go beyond them had made our sex life so predictable that it was half-dead. As we broke out of our established routines, I realized that this is how sexual ruts are formed: people limit themselves to the few safe moves they know and refuse to explore all that lies beyond their comfort zone.

These immature ways of dealing with our sexuality and the various pervasive mythologies about fairy-tale sex that overwhelm us in our youth persist for many people late into adulthood. We delude ourselves into thinking that real, enduring love is supposed to feel like the early space of falling in love. We naively expect our sexual lives to continuously be generated by that early spark of physical intensity, and we are disappointed when we have to begin to work for our passion. This also explains many of the premature endings that relationships suffer: we believe our attraction has died, when really it only needs to transform. We resist the idea that we are responsible for tapping into our own sexual desire and that no one else has the magic to make us feel sexy. Not only are we incapable physically of sustaining the intense, out-of-our-mind euphoria of early biological attraction, but also, more importantly, relying on that euphoria distracts us from the more mature forms of loving. Having the courage to grow up and become who we really are sexually, to discover our own capacity for arousal and make a safe haven in which to push our own boundaries, is how sex evolves into the amazing and transformative relationship-glue it is.

But it does take courage. When I think back on my husband's courage to offer me that first gift of lingerie and my own courage to accept it, I still wonder how it happened. I have asked him many times to explain to me what sparked that change. Nothing more, he says, than realizing things could be different, that he could have a great sex life. Maybe he felt like he had nothing to lose after the fifteen years of rejection and anger we had come to accept as normal. In this book I've talked a lot about knowledge, exploration, and education, and those things are indispensable. But in any relationship there are moments when you have to *do* something—something hard: you have to take a risk.

>> One courageous step that can make a big difference
in partnered sexual satisfaction is becoming
comfortable with masturbation. Even though
masturbation is the most common sexual act on the
planet, many people still struggle with accessing
their own pleasure. Overcoming our feelings of
shame associated with self-pleasure takes courage.

Yet masturbation is often referred to as the cornerstone of sexual pleasure, because when we learn our own pathways to our pleasure response, we not only gain a great sense of freedom in realizing that we are in control of our own pleasure, but also we greatly enhance our skills to share that pleasure response with our partner.

A good time to explore self-touch is in the shower or bath. Allow yourself to really feel your vagina, to explore the texture and folds of your labia and clitoris. Don't be afraid to put a finger inside your vagina and explore there, too. Move your hand over your entire genital area, noticing where the sensitive places are. Do the same with your breasts; play with your nipples. Your body belongs to you. Let yourself touch all of it without shame.

As you become more comfortable touching yourself alone, invite your partner to bathe with you. Begin just by watching each other touch your own bodies, so you can learn all the ways you each find pleasure. Then trade hands and let your partner guide your hand to all of their most erogenous zones.

The truest thing one can say about courage is that it is the ability to live well with all the risks that come with being human. We vacillate between the fear of living and the fear of dying, and in some ways our fears about our sexuality encompass both: we are terrified equally of opening up to our erotic fantasy life and of never fully experiencing the pleasure we know we contain in us. These fears strangle our capacity for intimacy and are the source of the harshest judgments we carry about the sexuality of others, even those we hold most dear. Whether they are instilled in us by early religious teachings or encoded and passed through our first family structure, our sexual fears take root when our erotic selves are just emerging. As we mature, these fears often become the deep and tragic inhibitions that prevent us from evolving sexually.

It is easy to feel helpless in the face of these fears and the inhibitions they create. They fit us so snugly that they become a second skin. It is hard to imagine a life without them or what kind of magical intervention we need to overcome them. But the courage to overcome your sexual inhibitions and fears is something that can be learned and practiced. Courage comprises four attributes: vulnerability, trust, resilience, and persistence. None of these four attributes is something you are just born with or something that comes to you magically; rather, each is developed and strengthened through practice.

As we explore these four attributes, we discover that our capacity to become courageous is about *cultivating a relationship to our fear*, not magically extinguishing it. Thinking of your inhibitions with this intent and asking yourself *how you listen to your fear* is a worthy beginning. Does your relationship to fear prevent you from doing the things you want to do? Do your fears create anxiety, so that you spend most of your energy worrying about them? Do you have the ability to witness your fear, make room for it, and work with it? Having and acting from a place of courage does not mean that our fears go away, but it does create the space where we can live more closely with what frightens us and engage with it. When my husband and I finally began the work of healing our sexual relationship, there was plenty of fear and anxiety. What changed wasn't our level of fear but our willingness to work with it.

Let's examine the development of courage with one of the most common and destructive issues for many long-term relationships, if not all—the question of who initiates. Looking at who in the relationship does most of the asking for sex, who does most of the rejecting, and the painful scorekeeping is a good place to practice courage. Becoming more courageous with the initiation question is a process that builds on itself, and it is a way out of the toxic shame and isolation that lead many couples to premature endings. Developing and strengthening the four attributes of courage within yourself through the initiation question is the key to healing your sexual relationship—both with your own desire and with your partner.

VULNERABILITY

Sexual desire issues are an integral part of long-term relationships. Everyone involved in a long-term relationship will face the issue of differing desires at some point, and often multiple times over the course of their relationship. In my own marriage, I have visited both sides of the desire fence. Although it has been suggested that the partner who refuses has more power in the relationship, my experience was that whichever side I was on, I felt powerless to stop the hurtful destruction this issue was wreaking on our relationship. Whether I wanted more intimacy and felt rejected or I did not want any intimacy at all, our relationship sustained the injuries. The potential for rejection got to be so painful that not asking at all became the discomfort zone we lived in. Like many people, I didn't fully understand all the meaning attributed to the initiation question; I knew only the shame and dwindling self-worth that seemed to suffocate me each time we talked about our sex life—or more often the lack of it. Sexual rejection is one of the deepest injuries we sustain, one that cuts to the core of how we perceive ourselves as worthy and desirable.

Over the years, I've come to see sexual desire as one of the most courageous forms of wanting. Because *desire is vulnerability*. We make ourselves vulnerable both in our wanting more intimacy and, even more deeply, in seeing ourselves as loveable. The vulnerability is intense, not only because we risk not getting what we want and experiencing rejection but also because being rejected by a life partner can wreak havoc on our perception of ourselves. Our sexual hunger is powerfully motivating in part because it carries so much risk. Our physical desire is one of the most powerful engines of self-fulfillment we are graced with.

And yet all desire is not created equal. When our longing for another comes from our perceived emotional weakness or lack of worthiness, it is driven by codependent need. Rather than making us more courageous, our longing then holds our partner and our relationship hostage. Conversely, when our desire springs from our best selves, in which we are emotionally self-aware and confident in our sexual longing, we have the courage to be curious, to take risks, and to expand beyond our previous experience. Healthy desire is not possessive or jealous. It doesn't drive us to try to control and change our partner but comes from a true longing for the other person, just as they are.

In my early twenties, I didn't have the courage to be vulnerable and risk this kind of wanting. I spent decades needing to be needed more than I could ever risk trusting that I could be wanted. This dynamic is a classic dilemma that often plays out in some form in many young relationships—the partner who won't or can't risk desire pairs with someone who won't or can't actively choose intimacy, and both then settle for circumstances where they don't ever have to risk longing or the possibility of rejection.

Many couples never find their way out of this desire conundrum and miss the simple yet essential step that makes desire truly authentic: the most critical aspect of wanting something is having the guts to choose it. Deliberate choices are the building blocks of self-creation. And yet committing to any choice is so difficult because it requires giving up all other possibilities. Many relationships struggle and wither because one or both partners are not able or willing to fully commit and choose their partner or relationship.

Desire that comes from conscious choice is potent. It carries the potential of real forgiveness, which allows the present to be different from the past. Passionate desire cannot be forced, cajoled, or manipulated; it must be chosen freely. This was the doorway to healing in my own relationship. Coming back to my desire without the fears and shame that had long been associated with it was one of the most liberating and courageous choices I have ever made. When I chose to accept the gift of lingerie from my husband, I was choosing desire, which meant choosing to stay vulnerable. If we hadn't chosen to stay vulnerable, our relationship would have ended, as many do.

Allowing ourselves to become truly vulnerable in the face of the difficult choices that define a mature, fulfilled life, and especially around all of the questions that deep intimacy provokes, is how our courage claims and grows the erotic soul. We mistakenly believe that we have to face our most challenging intimate moments with a kind of steely, unfeeling resolve, closing ourselves off to our feelings and, worse still, from the people we are closest to. Inadvertently, we carve out a life full of routines and habits to keep feelings of vulnerability at bay. We misinterpret vulnerability as a kind of weakness, instead of cultivating the power that comes from our most raw and authentic self. The more we resist and harden ourselves, the less open we are to what makes us most human and most capable of pleasure and intimacy. Our erotic selves require us to find comfort in vulnerability, just as the ability to let go is essential to our physiological capacity for orgasm.

TRUST

Trust is one of the basic building blocks in human relationships and one of the most fragile yet foundational aspects of shared sexuality. Real trust begins within us, when we believe in our own experience and choose our own thought process. Individuals without the ability for self-trust have trouble not only trusting others but also being trust-worthy. This dynamic plays itself out within our sexuality in pervasive and hurtful ways. Ironically, sexuality that is inhibited by a lack of self-trust shows up both as sexual frigidity and as various forms of pro-miscuity. When we don't trust our own judgment, we may believe we are breaking with our sexual fears and inhibitions by having uncom-mitted sex, but often we are inadvertently strengthening the fears that control us. Reckless sex, whether in hookups or affairs, is harmful to our ability to trust and be trusted because rather than moving us closer to what we really want—the deep love, acceptance, and release of fear that come with true sexual freedom—it keeps us isolated and alone with our fears.

Our attraction to this reckless sex comes from a persistent misper-ception about the nature of desire. Many of us still believe that sex is working only if it begins with a spontaneous eruption of desire, like when we fell in love and made out in the back seat of a Chevy with our first lover. That spontaneous fire is not only passionately intoxi-cating but also compelling because we are overcome by it. When sex happens to us in this out-of-control way, we don't have to be respon-sible for choosing it. Although getting swept up and overcome by our desire, especially illicit desire, may be the easiest route to arousal, it does not increase our ability to trust ourselves sexually, because we don't feel responsible for the choice. When we come to believe that the only access we have to our sexuality is when it overcomes us, we are teaching ourselves to devalue the trust and work required to create an ongoing sexual relationship.

This is problematic because over the course of a lifetime, the window of opportunity for our spontaneous sexual response is relatively brief. Our erotic desire only overwhelms us like this when we are deep in the throes of falling in love, when our biological and hormonal impulse to reproduce is fueling the engine. We wind up seeking illicit affairs to spark that uncontrollable combustion of carnal lust that is the only thing driving our sexual choices. The costs for relying on spontaneous desire are high. Sexual infidelity ranks as one of the top reasons cited for ending long-term relationships. Breaking sexual trust with those we love is for many an unforgiveable and unforgettable breach, and it rarely creates the foundation for long-term healthy relationship. Not only are most long-term relationships destroyed by the affair, the short-term, passion-based relationship also cannot survive. And a loss of trust tends to follow those who perpetuate the breakdown of relationships.

Building trust in our sexual life means rethinking our engagement with our erotic soul. Part of building this trust is being willing to surrender to the work of cocreating the spark, being willing to claim and be responsible for our own desire. Sex therapists refer to this more sustainable form of desire as "responsive," which means that it is generated by our intention and willingness to access our libido by becoming intimate and knowledgeable about our own arousal mechanism. By committing to find the sexual spark in ourselves, we learn to trust our own sexual response and, more importantly, to know that we have the ability to respond sexually when we choose to. Giving up the idea that you have to passively wait for your desire frees you up for all kinds of creative scheming and planning. And the more you practice accessing arousal and becoming a willing orchestrator of your own intimate moments, the more natural and easy it becomes. In fact, all the work of preparation starts to meld into the act of making love itself, and just like that, stirring the fire awake becomes an act of love toward both yourself and your partner. Learning how to get things going with your arousal mechanism will lead you back to the path of desire over and over, and there is nothing broken about this way in, except your willingness to do it.

As we begin to trust ourselves and our capacity for our own sexual choices, we also begin to trust our partner's right to have the same freedom to define sex for themself. So much of the dishonesty and judgment about what sex means comes from our inability to trust and be responsible for our own sexuality. Building sexual trust with your partner allows the dance of the erotic to unfold, choreographed not by any socially constructed ideas of sexuality, but by the tension of coming together and moving apart. Regardless of sexual preferences, this erotic dance is one of the most profound experiences of living in a body. It is the ultimate experience of letting go and holding on. Let your erotic self be the teacher, the guide, and the way to the momentary epiphanies that show us that the force of love is the guiding principle in the universe.

RESILIENCE

We cannot really be courageous without also becoming resilient. Resilience grows out of our increasing capacity to be vulnerable in our relationships and a dependable ability to trust ourselves. When we're resilient and we don't get what we want, we can take what we do get and work with it. Likewise, when we get what we believed we wanted but it turns out not to be what we expected, resilience gives us the courage to reexamine our desire and to ask questions about the gap between our expectations and reality. This is the process of sexual growth, of not giving up on our own capacity for desire. Resilience teaches us that if one thing doesn't work, something else will.

Resilience kicks in during the moments when life is falling apart. This deep inner work of rethinking and renegotiating is one of the highest forms of self-love. It is the effort that transforms us into our most authentic and compassionate selves. Certainly cultivating a mature sexual response deserves this kind of courage. When we are faced with adversity, the outcome has less to do with the external circumstances than it does with what we bring to the challenge from inside. How we transform all of life's challenges, and especially our sexual roadblocks, into something that makes us more whole is our capacity to not give ourselves away. Resilience is really a more radical kind of trust in ourselves, which keeps us present to the truth about ourselves and prevents us from making the situation worse with some familiar, downward-spiraling story line of victimization and blame.

Resilience, like love, is a seed of goodness that we all contain. It teaches us to befriend ourselves when things go wrong. As one of the highest forms of self-compassion, resilience backs us up and encourages us to try again. It encourages us to know and play to our strengths. We improve this skill through regular daily choices: by choosing foods that nourish us instead of junk or filler foods, by spending time with people who appreciate us instead of people who undermine us, by giving our attention to things that spark our curiosity and desire to know instead of getting lost in negative story lines that surround us in the news and on social media.

When it comes sexual courage, the most essential reason for building your own muscles of resilience is that it is the only way to ensure living in a resilient sexual relationship. Many a valuable relationship has been abandoned because one or both of the partners did not have the ability to see beyond their shared adversity and hold on to the many gifts that were also present. Resilience becomes more powerful when it is shared; having someone show up with true tenacity of spirit buoys us in even the darkest moments. All long-term, healthy sexual relationships rely on each partner's ability to believe in a future that might not always be apparent. This is the ultimate form of showing up for someone you love: having the courage to bear the disappointment of moments that don't work and the patience to tolerate the discomfort and not make the situation worse by spinning it into a story that cements everyone's pain.

Erotic resilience also encourages curiosity. The practice makes it easier to try different things, have them not work, and try again or try something new. A sexually resilient person can have experiences, even uncomfortable ones, without closing the door to experimenting. They have the ability to grieve and then move on after a relationship ends. In my work with couples, I've seen how many women become asexual early in their relationship—because they are not resilient, because they're afraid of their own desire, because they embrace their fears more than they embrace their relationship to fear. I've also worked with couples for whom the collateral damage of the initiation question and the feeling of not being desired by the other person has been the loss of their ability to respond sexually. This is where a capacity for resilience defines the direction of the relationship and in many ways of a life. Giving up has its own momentum and can overtake our thinking without our realizing that we have fallen into a path with no heart.

Having resilience brings a strong source of worthiness. Even when things are at their very worst, when you seem to be moving away from rather than toward realizing your desires, resilience can say, "Don't give up. You're worth it." You have the ability to hold yourself, even when nobody else will.

Finding resilient courage to think well of yourself when everything is broken is a gift. Developing the capacity to think well of yourself, even at the lowest moments, gives you the ground to think well of others, and this compassionate reciprocity of kindness and encouragement can often be the impetus that lets you turn the corner. It is an essential element in the health and longevity of any relationship. The most heroic stories we tell and the greatest love stories that get passed on through centuries share this one truth: that overcoming the odds with compassion, trust, and faith is the only story worthy of our efforts. You have everything you need to write your own heroic tale: trusting life begins with building your muscle of resilience.

PERSISTENCE

I remember going to a friend's wedding years ago, when I was just arriving at the end of my first decade of marriage. When I think back to that time in my marriage, mostly I remember how painful it was and how little was working. Our sex life was broken, there was no light on the horizon, and we were generally distant and estranged.

I remember asking myself why I kept staying. At the time, being married was work—the work of raising children, of managing our financial debt, of dealing with in-laws, and the really painful work of trying to sort out our sexual connection. Listening to my friend's vows, I remembered the promises that my husband and I had made to each other years before, and I realized again that where courage becomes real is in the action verb of persisting. It is the one aspect of courage that all the others rely upon, this ability to come back, again and again, to the pain and the discomfort to transform what is most difficult into something workable.

For most of us, this is the most difficult attribute of courage to develop. It requires strong discipline, and it also depends on the three other attributes for support. When things don't seem to be going well, pulling ourselves up again and again and telling ourselves that we're worth the effort takes resilience, trust that things will work out, and a willingness to stay vulnerable. But persistence is where the tire hits the road. It's not courage if you just do something brave one time, one day; it's only courage if you do it persistently.

All of the most important things that I care most deeply about in my life exist because I learned early not to quit, that by staying we make ourselves available to the change that is bound to come. Usually the moment when we think we can't stand it anymore is the moment when something shifts, the moment that makes sense of the struggle to get there.

Being persistent isn't about being stubborn and subjecting your-self to endless pain or suffering. Sometimes you can see that what you're doing is not working and hasn't worked in a long time. That's when it's time to change—not to give up, but try a fresh approach. And yet, even though you feel stressed, overwhelmed, unsatisfied, and doubtful about your present course or relationship, it is some-how easier to fall back on habit than to face the empty space of not knowing how to do it differently. You need to make a change but don't really know how to do it, so you watch yourself continuously go back to doing it the old way, the way you know.

Continuing with behaviors or relationships that we know deep down don't work or no longer fit in our life doesn't feel courageous. It feels like being stuck. *Insistence* can masquerade as *persistence*. The truth is that it takes a lot of work to change even a single habit that has developed a deep groove in us after years of reinforcement. How can we tell if the courageous action is to persist and work within the stuck place or to let go and reinvent? One clear way is to look at how present you are able to stay to your own experience. Often when we are stuck, we try to avoid our feelings and experiences. Allowing life to change and not staying with what is easy but unsatisfying takes a whole different kind of persistence and discipline.

Allowing yourself, your life, and your relationships to change and evolve, while giving yourself the time and space to figure out how to reinvent the situation, is the truly courageous act. Yet for many of us, facing the unknown is so uncomfortable that we opt for the often harder but predictable banging of the head against the wall. Seeing the difference between these spaces requires our fullest attention. Having the courage and willingness to embrace these moments of deep questioning and to live inside of them sufficiently is what allows the answers to emerge. Choosing to persist with the discomfort and ambivalence of not knowing instead of continuously reverting to our old ways is always courageous.

Couples locked into old habits of communication, or lack of it, or those trapped in troubled, repetitive intimacy cycles know what is wrong. They don't need a therapist to tell them where things aren't working. They just don't know how to do it right. Confronting honestly what is broken and having the courage to embrace the space of transition takes real courage. Persisting in the face of the unknown may be one of the most courageous acts of all. The painful yet familiar habits can call back to you and feel comforting as you make your way in the dark. This is when the capacity to remain vulnerable, to trust in a process that you cannot direct, and to be resilient in self-compassionate friendship allows the courageous will of persistence to guide you to create something new and workable.

>> Choose a sexual fear that you have never had the courage to deal with. It could be a sexual act you have always wondered about or overcoming shame about being sexual in the body you have. Write down a sexual goal related to this fear and share it with your partner or a trusted friend. Living inside the vulnerability of this exposure may be uncomfortable at first, so choose your confidante wisely so that you can also expand your ability to trust in this exposed space. Create a detailed action plan with a timeline of steps that will expand your exploration of new sexual experiences, making them progressively challenging. Increasing the challenge will test your resilience, and following through on a number of steps will teach you the way of persistence—not just sexually, but in every way.

As eagles prepare to mate, they lock talons and free-fall through the sky. It is a do-or-die proposition—as it is with us humans. Each time we take a leap to live our authentic lives and throw ourselves forward, with heart wide open, we are cultivating our relationship to fear. How we respond to what frightens us is, in essence, how we respond to the whole of our lives. The more we cultivate the skills that make us courageous—being vulnerable, trusting ourselves, practicing resilience, and learning persistence—the more we build our capacity for the next challenge. Fear begets fear, and courage begets courage.

Martin Luther King Jr. wrote this about fear: "Normal fear protects us; abnormal fear paralyses us. Normal fear motivates us to improve our individual and collective welfare; abnormal fear constantly poisons and distorts our inner lives. Our problem is not to be rid of fear but rather to harness and master it."[1] Bringing this idea of harnessing and mastering our fears into our relationships and our sexuality provides them with the space to blossom into deeply fulfilling sources of self-recognition and pleasure. Courageous relationships encourage both partners to experiment and grow. Facing life challenges with the courage to see that we *do* always have choices and practicing the skills to choose in favor of life rather than fear, we find ourselves in a life we can love, a life of our own making.

5

CURIOSITY

Perhaps the single most overlooked attribute that has the potential to transform a life is curiosity. An inborn trait that defines us as small children, curiosity is our eagerness to explore, our desire to know and understand our world and ourselves, and our urge to go beyond our own limits. As the mother of four, I have witnessed over and over how little I actually taught my children and how much of their development was really about me keeping them safe while they followed their own curiosity. Curiosity is the seed of wonder in us. When we befriend this wonder and offer it our full attention, it will guide our awareness to what we are not seeing, providing meaningful questions to help us know ourselves and the world. It predicts our capacity to learn, change, and adapt.

Our social network and the depth of the relationships within that network exist in proportion to our curiosity. Remember the Sexual Identity Grid? How isolated we feel on that grid has a lot to do with our capacity for curiosity. As adults, we often lose sight of the expansive and curative practice of following our curiosity and discovering the world, both outside of us and in our own souls. Imperceptibly, our curiosity is replaced with judgment, spurred by unnamed fears, and this separates us from our own experience as well as the people closest to us. Fortunately, like courage, our capacity for curiosity is developmental, which means that it can grow when given the opportunity.

Let's face it: what we are most attracted to in someone, given enough time, usually becomes repulsive to us. It is an odd but insistent phenomenon that characterizes most intimate relationships. When it began to happen early in my marriage, I was unprepared for the intensity with which my loving attraction became infused with judgment, impatience, and disdain. Michel had taught me a lot about sex, but I still had a lot to learn about how to sustain a relationship. I had known all along the man I was going to marry was the strong, silent type. We even built the idea of protecting each other's solitude into our vows. But I didn't understand how his comfort with silence and quiet would provoke all my old feelings of loneliness. And the lonelier I felt in my marriage, the more distant I became sexually as well.

I am sure that this contributed to the deep sexual divide we experienced, where keeping score of who asked and who said no only increased the emotional distance that became the flip side of our strong attraction. When this happens, most of us don't recognize that we have been letting our curiosity about the other person slowly be replaced with judgments.

Esther Perel's best-selling work *Mating in Captivity* describes this phenomenon, which often evolves into the deadening of passion that happens over time in long-term relationships. One of the key reasons she cites is the conflict-averse culture in which most of us are raised, training couples to become more like each other over time and less like themselves.[1] In our efforts to avoid the inevitable conflicts that come from recognizing and living with our differences, we give up what makes us most uniquely ourselves—which is the intrigue that made the erotic sparks fly to begin with. Worse still, the more of ourselves we give up to be in a partnership, the more resentful we become, often without even realizing it. Our attraction to the other is replaced slowly with a repulsion that we don't understand and cannot articulate, gradually eroding how authentically we engage.

This is what had happened to my husband and me. His neat and orderly qualities, which were once so endearing, drove me crazy. My impulsive and creative musings became grating instead of inspiring. We weren't unusual. This is the course of love over time. Often, as couples experience the flip side of what they once loved, they try to get back there by giving up those parts of themselves that have become the source of conflict. It is easy to see how this happens: no one wants to lose the warm, loving connection that pulled them into their relationship, so we call it compromise, the giving up of the qualities that make us so uniquely ourselves.

Sadly, this is a losing strategy that usually ends up, as Perel describes, in a passionless and sexless marriage where no one risks being authentically themselves. This is why many people experience the feeling of coming back to themselves once they have left their partner, whether temporarily or permanently.

One quality that all long-term passionate lovers share is their dedication to remaining two deeply individuated people who are committed to living with their differences, even when those differences create conflict. The courage to hold on to our selves as we move deeper into our relationships becomes the rudder by which we steer. Honoring our individuality offers both the clarity of negotiating conflict and the fuel of passionate connection. So even as we experience the inevitable cycles of attraction and rejection, we hold fast to the essence of our own being. As we gain more experience with these cycles, we see how they form the energetic patterns of moving together and apart, creating waves that spark intrigue and excitement, renewing our curiosity for each other and keeping our relationship alive.

The best couples therapist that we ever saw, Bob, taught us this secret when our relationship was most volatile and hurtful. Both of us were struggling to hold on to our selves while figuring out how to get back to appreciating the differences in the other. By this time, my resentment of my husband was so overwhelming, I felt like it swallowed me whole. I remember Bob asking me to hold out one hand as I was burning with furious tears.

"Okay, Wendy," he said. "Your feeling of resentment is in this hand. Now open the other hand. Remember when he showed up for you last, when he was tender with you even when you were angry."

Mature love happens when you can hold those hands open side by side, when you realize that someone can be both what you love and what you hate simultaneously. Over the years, this lesson has not only enabled my husband and me to cultivate a mature, evolving capacity for love, but it has also contained the seed of passionate intimacy.

One of the most primary acts of growing up is learning to live with the split between what we like and what we don't like. Over time, it becomes clear that our likes and dislikes often prevent us from seeing who is in front of us. This recognition is the beginning of slowly replacing judgment with curiosity and coming to understand that our greatest strengths are also our greatest weaknesses. As we become more comfortable with the terrain of light and dark and how they are always simultaneously at play inside each of us, we learn how to love in a more mature way. In doing this, we also become forgiving. Because we know this truth to be universal, it gets easier to work with how the parts of us that were once so attractive can also be, at times, so annoying.

Learning how to claim this space of individuation and acceptance is a practice that requires both discipline and curiosity. Giving up our emotional reactivity takes practice. We need both impulse control and the ability to distance ourselves from our familiar knee-jerk reactions. Instead of acting on the feelings of attraction and repulsion that arise from our differences, we learn to wrap our initial emotional response in *curiosity*. First we work to stop taking our partner's behavior personally—it becomes clear that our partner's differences are not about us—and then we have the space to open up to wonder what drives them to act, think, and behave the way they do.

As we cultivate our curiosity and grow stronger in our commitment to understanding our erotic self, the container of our relationship becomes stronger, which in turn allows our curiosity to roam further and freer. By learning to hold our capacity for attraction and rejection side by side, we create more spaciousness and authenticity in our sexual relationship. This mature form of love makes your heart bigger and more capable of expressing compassion and listening deeply, which are essential skills for passionate union. Creating the space that allows your partner to be who they are allows you to witness and feel their efforts to love you more truly.

Our erotic soul, the purest and rawest part of our humanity, needs judgment-free space to unfold. In the vast spectrum of our life experience, both achieving the freedom to release orgasmic sexual energy and transforming the push-pull of love and hatred into an open jungle of potential passion begin with curiosity about why and how we could be so different and still want to eat each other up.

Relationships are the natural incubators of our curiosity. Just as the parent-child relationship creates a safe environment through which children can explore the world, adult relationships can become the ideal laboratories for fostering adult curiosity. An intimate relationship provides the safe container for us to explore the most intimate human experiences, from powerful emotions to the eroticism of the body. And in the same way that unsupervised children are at a greater risk of harm than lovingly supervised children, we adults are more likely to get hurt—and to hurt others—when we explore our emotional and erotic world without the protective embrace of loving, respectful relationships.

The beauty of cultivating our sense of curiosity in our relationships is that it reinforces itself in a vital and self-perpetuating cycle. Our curious explorations make our relationships stronger and more open, and as a relationship changes and grows, it invites more and more curiosity from us. Curiosity is a natural ally of freedom, especially sexual freedom. Allowing our curiosity to roam freely is an enlightening and inherently sexy process, because adding wonder—without judgment—makes relationships more spacious, inviting in the unknown and opening us to places that have yet to be discovered. Your judgment-free curiosity will be contagious, providing your partner with the permission, even encouragement, to explore in a new way.

The ability to give your partner the space to become more of themself is a gift you really give yourself, especially when it comes to sex. For most of us, our erotic selves are the least developed and most mysterious parts of who we are. If you are busy trying to become more like someone else or trying to control some part of who you are that sets off a bad reaction in someone else, you shut down the sense of safety necessary to access and explore who you are erotically. When the love container of your relationship is strong enough to hold your differences without threat of reprisal or rejection, then the wild side of your erotic self has space to come out and play. This is where our differences become intriguing and can once again ignite passion.

Becoming more curious also allows us to become more vulnerable. That's why, in many ways, creating safe space for curiosity is the antidote to our fear. When our desire to know trumps our fear of being seen, we are emboldened to venture into the unknown and otherwise frightening territory of sexual exploration. My husband's gift of lingerie unleashed in me a torrent of desire and fantasies, and I was swept away by the wildness of my sexual curiosity, which I had been suppressing for so long.

My curiosity allowed me to finally begin looking at those fantasies—and I was terrified. For most of us, fantasies are rarely politically correct. Mine were full of deep, subconscious stuff that troubled me. Where did they come from? It was hard to believe I could imagine these fantasies, let alone talk about them with anyone. And so, at the moment my husband and I were finally finding the courage to open up sexually, I began to shut down. The fantasies feeding my passion felt so taboo that my fear overcame my curiosity. I didn't know how to be comfortable with this fantasy life inside of me.

It was deeply troubling. I knew that if I couldn't remain open to my own fantasy life, there would be an expanse of passion that I would never have access to. Luckily for me, during this time I was working hard to remain curious about my erotic self. I was also hosting a radio show that brought me into conversations with sex therapists, psychologists, and spiritual healers. Stanley Siegel, one of the authors I had the opportunity to speak to, had just published a book about sexual fantasy, and in my conversation with him, I learned many things about human fantasy lives that, in turn, made me more curious about myself. Like most positive attributes we cultivate, curiosity allows for more curiosity. When we develop the habit of being curious in our relationships, it soon comes to shape the way we engage with our lives. That single conversation gave me permission to get to know my previously repressed fantasy life, which turned out to be rocket fuel for passionate intimacy. Had I turned away from my curiosity at that moment, I would have never learned the most important lesson I have ever gained about growing up sexually, and I would have lost the vital sense of wonder that continues to keep me young.

As I found the gateway to my own curiosity, three things became clear to me. First, I learned that our curiosity is fragile. It can be silenced by our fears and the limitations we impose on ourselves to remain "safe." By trying to avoid things that trouble us, we unwittingly put up walls to knowing ourselves. And like most self-imposed limits, these walls don't just block our curiosity about that one thing—they block all of our wonder. We get stuck in what we refuse to see. Boredom is a sorry substitute for experience.

Second, I learned that once you believe something isn't accessible to you, it actually becomes inaccessible. Ever notice how it's impossible to have an orgasm when you're worrying about whether it will or won't happen? Our anxiety and the self-imposed, protective limitations inhibit our curiosity and ability to connect. Without the magic of curiosity we become isolated, not just from others but also from ourselves.

And, maybe most importantly, I learned that there is nothing to fear when it comes to true sexual curiosity. Even my wildest and most disturbing fantasies, acted out consensually and causing no harm, are there to teach my husband and me and to free us to an ever greater capacity for pleasure. If ever there was a place in life to allow our curiosity free rein, it is in the realm of erotic exploration. By giving myself the freedom to learn about my fantasy life, an entirely new realm of sexual experience was opened to me.

Nothing undermines curiosity faster than disapproval and fear. Sadly, many of us had our innate childhood curiosity squelched before we even noticed it was there. When the messages we grow up hearing mostly begin with "no" and "don't," our curiosity is pushed underground. When we are not safe to wonder, to question, to get dirty looking for answers, we are effectively being taught to close ourselves off to much of the world.

A child's mind that is run by fear of disapproval and loneliness is trapped. Its thinking is slowed and its capacity for wonder, limited. In retreat, the child's mind turns inward, away from the vast possibilities of life, and thoughts get caught in repetitive and unhealthy patterns, like a hamster on a wheel. Instead of seeking out new people and new ideas, the mind gets primed in fear and judgment, slowly shutting down to the wonder of being alive.

Boredom is a symptom of a mind that has lost its way, that has no active mechanism to reach beyond itself. Lacking curiosity over time, we lose access to our imagination. We become passive receptacles for easily available entertainment. We become dependent on all forms of media to fill us and to occupy our time. Screen time becomes a kind of addiction—one that brings increasingly less satisfaction. We require more and more intense stimulation to fend off the feeling of wasting time and spinning our wheels. But it is nothing like the pure urge of creativity and aliveness that happens when we follow our curiosity. Curiosity is active, creating the urge to do and to discover. It is the process by which we discover ourselves and wake up our intrinsic motivation. It also inherently teaches us how to respond to change. With curiosity we can adapt both to external circumstances and our own growth. Without curiosity we lose the ability to imagine living our lives differently.

One of the places where our lack of curiosity and imagination takes the biggest toll is in our sexual lives. Many of us are so terrified to open up to the mystery of our sexuality that our fear actually shuts down our libido altogether. We long for a sexually passionate response but are unable to imagine ourselves outside our comfort zone. Without sexual curiosity, we cannot imagine and ask for what we want, and without knowing our own pleasure response, we accept cheap imitations—packaged goods ready for easy download—which only stifle our curiosity more. Without access to our curiosity, we become numb, which explains the epidemic of people who heavily self-medicate and still cannot feel anything sexually.

Here's the amazing thing about curiosity: choosing to become more curious in any area of life will positively impact all the other areas, including sex. Practicing the art of curiosity—opening the mind while staying fully present—will change the landscape, both in the bedroom and out. Becoming more curious and open-minded about what happens to you during the day will also change what happens in your bedroom. Next time you hit a roadblock, start asking yourself questions. Seek out and experiment with new flavors and scents, and take time to really process the sensations on your tongue and in your nose. Scent and taste are some of the most visceral experiences where we can observe curiosity in action.

There are a ton of best sellers supporting the ideas that monogamy kills sexual passion and that sexual boredom is inevitable in long-term relationships. Equally popular and detrimental to many a sex life is the belief that sexual attraction, or the degree of passionate chemistry in a relationship, is a viable indicator of the health of the relationship. This same mythology populates movies and television: great sex lives don't take work; they just happen to you. Furthermore, the mythology says you shouldn't have to plan for sex; in fact, planning takes the zest away. We are taught to expect our passion to fade, so when it does, we accept it as inevitable. We aren't even curious about why the passion has disappeared.

The key to seeing through this mythology is understanding and embracing a fundamental truth: your curiosity about your own sexuality and your willingness to understand and explore it can make sex really hot. The moment you bring wonder into the sexual equation, you take responsibility for your own desire and arousal, and you discover the rare and magical freedom to make a sex life that works. Hitting the wall of sexual boredom with your partner is actually a clear message that your relationship is ready and wanting to grow and expand. Becoming accustomed to each other and following the pleasure pathways you each routinely respond to should inspire you to question and try something else. Being open to change and seeking novelty in your sexual encounters spring from an authentic, loving desire to know yourself and your partner better.

Many long-term relationships fall into the space where our sexual repertoire is limited by the things we are afraid to try, or what sex therapist David Schnarch refers to as "leftover sex"—the sex that exists in the narrow range of sexual behaviors we are accustomed to. It can't help but get boring, and worse, it can lead couples to believe that they are sexually incompatible. Our lack of curiosity sits at the core of our sexual boredom, the most frequently cited reason for sexual affairs. What drives sexual restlessness has less to do with you or your partner and more to do with the nature of your partnership.

Sexual compatibility is often misunderstood as the union of two people with the same sexual appetite and comfort level; in actuality, lasting sexual compatibility is better defined as the union of two people who are both interested, curious, and flexible enough to stretch into wanting to know more about their partner's arousal. This is why having a sex life that works over time requires effort. In this way, lasting sexual passion is no different from—and, in fact, is a mirror for—the other work you do in your relationship. The emotional intimacy you cultivate in dealing with the rest of your life is exactly what will help you communicate about things that are difficult to articulate, like your sexual desires and fantasies.

Next time you are bored, ask questions. Dare yourself to get active and do something new. Look for the small things about your partner that make you wonder. Better still, try to do just one thing with or for your partner that makes you wonder why you never did it before.

>> Here are a few easy ways to shake up the world of leftover sex—simple things that might not push you into something totally new, but are new enough to make sex feel really different.

Change the time of day when you have sex. If it is always dark, try dusk. A little afternoon delight can make you feel like you stepped into a new movie. Within the sexual act itself, try changing the tempo. Go slow and deep, or fast and shallow, or mix it up.

Shake up your foreplay routine. Seduce your partner in another room of the house. (Eating at your kitchen table might never mean the same thing again.) Wash your partner in the shower—use a soapy hand as a preview of what is to come. Start before you even get into the house: while you're parked in the garage, take off your seat belts and let your bodies touch.

Buying something new, like lingerie or a vibrator, can be fun too, but don't rely on the new item to get your sexual juices flowing. Having great sex is a result of changes we make in our thinking, beliefs, and willingness to explore; it doesn't depend on new clothes or gadgets. Continuously opening up and searching for access to sexual pleasure takes work, but it may well be the most rewarding use of your creative powers.

Sexual curiosity diminishes or grows in tandem with our ability to communicate with our partner about our erotic self. Many people can't use words like *masturbate* in front of their partners, let alone share in the act together. When we don't embrace and communicate our fears about our sexual selves, they end up feeling like a small cage in which physical intimacy shrinks.

Asking questions of our fears is the first and best response. You cannot force your fears to respond, but inviting them into a conversation—and, more importantly, being willing to listen to your fears and internal judgments—is often the beginning of thawing out a physical connection that has become frozen in silence over time. When our sexual curiosity is at its best, it increases our capacity to communicate. Wanting to know more about your erotic self and giving space for your sexual impulses builds connection and inspires experimentation.

Without communication, we become isolated, and isolation is an instant on switch for our fears and an off switch for our curiosity. When we don't express ourselves or allow ourselves to know our desires, our lives become smaller, and we are constrained. And yet, for many of us, feeling isolated and alone with our sexuality is standard. Learning how to communicate and express ourselves is not an inborn skill; we learn to do so as we expand our vocabulary and have opportunities to ask questions and formulate ideas.

Sadly, the formal sexual education that some of us received in our childhood and early adolescence was, at its best, an exercise in naming body parts, with genders separated in different rooms. We learned early to feel shame about this curiosity. Still today, much of "sex ed" is an oxymoron, replacing factual information with heavy doses of disease, abstinence, and sin. The truth is, we were all seriously undereducated and even, depending on our background, deliberately misinformed about our sexual selves and the acts of creating pleasure in loving, healthy ways.

For a long time, I could not talk to my husband about the new fantasies that came through me while we had sex. Ironically, the more intense and intimate our sex became, the less I could open up and share the shocking story lines and images that emerged in my mind as we were making love. It was vital at this point in my sexual development that I open up to learning more about what was happening to me. At that time, I was fortunate and so grateful to have my radio show, where I interviewed various sex experts and was gaining new, broader language for understanding and expressing all these previously unexplored and unnamed parts of myself. Education is always the most appropriate response when it comes to our curiosity. I have always believed that any question a child is mature enough to formulate begs an honest answer, because the child is capable of learning the truth. This holds true for the developing places in adult sexuality as well: acquiring the language with which we can understand and talk about our sexual experience enables us to share it, making it more authentic and trustworthy.

Taking control of our sexual education is one of the most loving acts we can do for our relationship with both our erotic self and our partner. One way that we can show respect for our curiosity is to seek out reliable sources of information. Sometimes this process might be as simple as asking questions and accepting feedback from our partners. But sometimes, as it was in my case, it might mean going out and seeking input from experts. There are many deeply skilled sexual health educators and therapists who have been invaluable in helping people grow up sexually. In the "Further Reading and Resources" section of this book, you'll find a list of books I've found immensely helpful in showing me how much there is to know about our sexual potential. These books are written by some of the most articulate sex therapists and educators I have met. They aren't only educational; I've included them because they're well-written and entertaining, too. The more we allow ourselves the guidance and information we need to trust our evolving sexual experiences, the more empowered we will feel.

There is probably no more important place to begin this erotic education than with our knowledge about our sexual anatomy, which remains remarkably misunderstood and the source of many issues that plague so many couples. When we don't fully understand how or why something happens inside of us, then communicating about it seems impossible. It is no wonder that our sexual skills are also often compromised.

In a recent *Men's Health* survey of five thousand men and women, 20 percent of women rated their partner's sexual skills as average or worse. Yet over 25 percent of women have never given their partner any feedback on his skills for fear of hurting his feelings. This is a shame considering that when men were asked about their openness to sexual feedback, fully 80 percent said, "Whatever you want.

All you have to do is ask." An additional 17 percent were open to feedback if she's "nice about it." Only 3 percent say they don't want to hear anything. Of the women who have given their men sexual advice, over 64 percent of them said that when they gave their partners feedback on their love skills, they experienced more pleasure; the same was true for nearly 60 percent of men.[2]

>> How little we know—and how much we assume— about our own partner's experience of sex can be surprising. A way to see this is to make a list of all the questions you've ever wanted to ask your partner about their sexual experience. Your list could include questions about their early sexual education and erotic lessons, their first sex experiences, and their fantasies. To learn more about their erogenous zones, you might ask, "How does it feel when I . . . ?" You could ask how they like to touch themselves when they're alone. Add everything to your list that makes you curious about the person you're most intimate with.

Then, when you're alone and relaxed together, ask your partner one of the questions from your list. As your partner opens up, notice the quality of your listening: curiosity makes us both more interested and more interesting.

One game that my husband and I have played many times when we needed to reset and that I have shared with many clients is a sexy version of "hot or cold." Borrowing from the popular children's game, use no words except *hot, warm,* and *cold* to direct your partner to the places you most enjoy being touched. Take ten- to fifteen-minute turns.

Simply by turning communication into a game, you increase the suspense and anticipation of play.

Be open to the pleasant surprises of the many unexplored erogenous zones you discover along the way. Love demands that we continuously rediscover the other and our relationship.

When I was younger, I was certain that someday I would reach a point where my life would stop changing. I would have turned over all the stones, seen all there was to see, figured things out. I never envisioned that at fifty-five I would still be turning over new stones in my marriage and sex life, that these things would still be changing all the time.

Some of the changes are still scary—like when I began menopause. For years prior, I was afraid that the disappearance of my hormones would impact my ability to orgasm. I had been easily orgasmic my whole life, and I was anxious after hearing stories from menopausal women about their increasing disinterest in sex and inability to orgasm. What would menopause mean for both my sex life and my marriage? Facing the end of the reproductive cycle that I knew as myself, I recall sharing my fears with my husband, wondering how we would manage.

Following my own prescription, I have expanded my reading and discovered other stories from women whose sex lives expanded and improved after menopause. I was encouraged to find that some women actually had more sexual energy after menopause and became curious about how their new body would create entirely new sensations. Although the changes that menopause has brought to my body means I can't rely on what used to "work" to help me climax, I have learned to trust that these new sensations can take me to a deeper and entirely new capacity for pleasure.

Because we never stop changing, there is always a need for curiosity. Curiosity keeps our senses alive and our minds young. When we stop being curious, we stop paying attention, and without our attention, we can live together with others yet still feel cut off, isolated, and alone. Sex that really works depends on keeping our capacity for discovery vital. This is also the key to lifelong learning and the ability to make different choices given the same stimulus. When you think you've answered all of the questions, just wait—something new *will* happen.

6

SENSATION

The journey of learning to feel depends on our deliberate intention to awaken our senses. Learning to slow down enough to live inside of our sensory capacities is both the meaning of and the path to true embodiment. There are no shortcuts to engaging through our senses. Getting back into the body isn't always pleasant or easy; in fact, sometimes confronting our weakest places is downright frightening. And the confrontation doesn't always happen according to our schedule. In my case, it took me completely by surprise.

Just as my curiosity was beginning to wake me up to the real erotic possibilities in my marriage, I badly injured my back. I was thirty-seven years old and had just had my fourth child. I still remember the moment it happened: all I did was turn, a disc slipped, and suddenly I was in excruciating pain. I lay on the floor, unable to get up, not knowing what I was going to do.

I was afraid of how debilitating this injury was and of how my body barely felt like my own. I had three young children and a newborn to raise, I didn't have time to be injured, and I didn't have time to deal with my body. And yet pain is a powerful teacher and will force you back into your body like nothing else. In many ways, I think of that injury as a crucial turning point in my erotic journey. Without it, I may have never learned a powerful lesson: that a life of pleasure demands a strong and agile core.

It might seem strange that pain can show us the next step toward sex that works, but the value of pain is that it calls our attention back to our bodies.

In confronting our pain and truly healing ourselves, we have to live fully in our bodies, because it is only through the body that we can discover the basis of erotic pleasure: our senses.

Before I was stopped in my tracks by my back pain, I would have said that my senses were doing fine—I could see and hear and smell just like anyone else. But I didn't realize how blunt and deadened they had become, because I had been ignoring my body for so long. Except for running after kids, I hadn't exercised in years. As I began to turn my situation around, I learned that my back was unbelievably weak because I had virtually no core strength. I relied on an elastic brace that I wore around my hips to hold me together. That degree of weakness seems like the kind of thing you would notice, but the truth is that once we check out of feeling our body, we have to be hit over the head with a brick to wake up again. This explains the rampant abuse of pharmaceutical painkillers, too: it gets easier and easier not to feel and to lose touch with your body. We push away the pain and discomfort for so long that turning back toward what is happening begins to feel impossible. In my case, I had been racing around for years meeting the needs of others while ignoring my own needs, distracting myself from all the ways that my body was weak.

But after that day when the pain immobilized me, I could no longer choose distraction. Hurting my back so badly presented me with a choice: I could battle my way back into my body and get strong, as difficult and painful as that was going to be, or I could curl up and medicate. For me it actually wasn't a choice; I knew I had to draw on my courage and decide to accept pain as a part of healing and moving toward pleasure.

After recuperating for some time in bed (thank God I had a doula), I began investigating exercise options. I knew I was out of shape, but when I started a Pilates class I was shocked to find out just how weak my core had actually become. Pilates was the perfect rehabilitation program. Because its carefully calculated, refined movements are targeted to make you feel into and understand each and every muscle, I could finally understand where the weakness started. Working through this weakness and the pain of getting stronger was the most challenging part of reclaiming my erotic self. I'm not sure I could have stayed with it if I hadn't also begun to notice the ways in which becoming fully present in my body during Pilates was also training me to be more present in my body at other times—like during sex. The work of strengthening all the connecting muscles in my pelvic floor was teaching me how to activate them, how to open them up to pleasure as well as pain. My husband noticed the change, too: the core muscles I was developing in class let me hold on to him with new strength. Our sex life was invigorated as I rediscovered all the sensations that come with stronger embodiment.

This reawakening of my physical strength encouraged my sexual curiosity to expand. Being strong is more *interesting* than being weak. I started paying more attention to my body and to the full range of sensations it was capable of—and each new sensation fueled my curiosity about what other sensations I could feel. Strength inspires not only curiosity but also daring. As we grow stronger, we trust ourselves to risk more.

Still, despite the core strength I was developing, there were ways in which my body, after four children, could not keep up with my curiosity. As sex became more interesting and passionate, I still didn't recover the biological capacity to self-lubricate. I was always very dry, even when I was intensely aroused—a very common side effect after pregnancy and nursing.

But this persistent dryness, like my back injury before it, turned out to be a blessing in disguise, as it forced me to pay attention and ask questions about what was happening. The dryness made me begin to investigate the whole process of lubrication. On my doctor's recommendation, I went searching for lubricants that would help with the persistent pain with sex that comes from insufficient lubrication. I purchased dozens of bottles from pharmacies and even went to adult stores. But every one I tried left me burning, awake, and in pain after sex. So while I soaked in the tub for an hour, my husband drifted off to sleep (which did not help our marriage). As I later learned, all of those lubricants were made of heavily concentrated petrochemical ingredients, which are toxic to that most sensitive genital tissue and are now known to disrupt the body's natural immune response, highly increasing the risk of many sexually transmitted diseases in addition to other unpleasant side effects.

I stepped up my efforts, looking everywhere and anywhere for a better lubricant, anything that would make sex fun again and not create all the nasty side effects. One day, browsing the shelves of a local shop, I found a little bottle of oil on closeout. When we used it later that night, I was overjoyed. Not only did it *not* create the terrible itching and burning of all the petrochemical lubricants, but also something else happened: the scent and the glide created some of the wildest pleasure I had shared with my husband in a very long time. Voila! We were back in business!

It wasn't until we ran out of the bottle of love oil and our sex life took a serious tumble that I realized what had really lit my fire was not just the ease and glide but also the *scent*.

I went back to the store, looking for another bottle, but they no longer carried the product. This time my searching became a little more desperate. I wanted that kind of sex again, but I couldn't find anything that would work as powerfully for us. Eventually I learned more about that first bottle of love oil and started mixing up essential oil formulations of my own, trying to recreate the scent that had driven me wild.

Working with essential oils awakened a whole new level of olfactory sensibility for me, and I became curious about the sense of smell itself. What was the powerful link to my arousal? How is it that a single smell can immediately summon distant memories, transporting us to a different time and place? As I pursued answers to my questions about the mystery of scent, I uncovered a huge body of research demonstrating the profound links between our capacity for smell and arousal. Our olfactory bulb, which processes scent, is co-located with our limbic brain, which is where we process memory, emotion, and sexuality. It wasn't surprising to learn that in ancient times, aphrodisiac oils were more valuable than gold.

I was all the more intrigued, and my collection of aromatherapy books and oils quickly expanded. I was experimenting with new combinations every day. Soon I had more love oil samples than I knew what to do with and started giving them away to family and friends. I knew from many of my friends and mothers of my children's classmates that I was not alone in struggling with my libido and pain with sex. As happens with many entrepreneurs, necessity became the mother of invention. It wasn't long before I founded my company, Good Clean Love, where I am evolving the use of aphrodisiac love oils and healthy personal lubricants to this day.

It's hard to believe that my journey of learning how to feel began with that first, life-stopping back injury, but that's what it took to finally get back into my body. And getting back into my body meant getting back into a world of sensation—and then that little bottle of love oil showed me the true erotic power of the sensory world. Learning to smell was the life-changing discovery that catapulted me into the wonder of my senses and revolutionized my access to the erotic. What I've found is that as our senses become more acute and we learn to train our attention on the plentiful rich textures that our senses give to life, everything is more erotic.

Yet, as I said at the start of this chapter, there is no quick and easy path on this journey of learning to feel. What I discovered is that feeling our way into our body and sensing our world requires a different kind of attention and demands that we get out of our heads. This can be daunting for many of us because we have spent so much time ignoring, medicating, and otherwise masking messages from our bodies. We have to learn again how to listen to those messages, as difficult as they may be to hear, and how to trust what we are feeling.

While coming back into our body makes us confront our own weaknesses, living inside of our own fragility also offers access to a wide range of sensory experience that we may have long ignored. Had my back injury not forced me to wake up to where I was weakest, I may have never become so intimate with my senses. I would have never discovered how the fragrance of early spring Daphne can completely change my mood or how other spicy scents can completely reinvent my arousal mechanism. During this time I also realized how much *looking* I had been doing for much of my life without really *seeing*. Our capacity for pleasure, sexual and otherwise, is enhanced and increased by our attention to our sensory input. As we learn to experience life through the sensory data that makes our memories more memorable and our life richer, we find ourselves living differently because we aren't just thinking, we are *feeling our experiences*.

The process of opening to our bodies begins with learning to focus our attention on the visceral sensations we are experiencing in each moment. It takes practice to move from looking to actually seeing, from hearing to the deeper capacity of listening, from consuming food to actually tasting and smelling it. In the rest of this chapter, we will explore how to practice this sensory awakening in the smallest of moments and how doing so steadily translates into feeling into the erotic.

This practice has been a cornerstone of my own erotic awakening. The more I learned to re-engage with my innate sensory capacities, the more I could awaken to my erotic impulses. You can't have an awakened sexual experience while living outside of your body; pleasure depends on your ability to feel what's happening to you from the inside. And once you do start to feel, everything is different. The world is much richer than you ever realized, the textures of life are more plentiful than you imagined, and your capacity to be sexual is more expansive than you knew.

Touch is the first language we learn and the only truly universal communication that humans share. Yet it is still not uncommon for parents to stop hugging their kids as they reach puberty. And for many adults, the physical nurturing we receive declines as we age, even as medical studies confirm that the health benefits of physical touch extend throughout our lives.

We have known for decades that babies who are not held and touched regularly do not thrive; the lack of physical contact is as harmful to their development as a lack of food. Skin-to-skin contact between babies and their mothers is now the standard of care in neonatal units worldwide because of its healing impact. Studies in orphanages demonstrate the same conclusions: babies who are given more physical touch develop better and get sick less often.[1]

It isn't just in babies that the power of touch transforms emotional, mental, and physical health. People suffering from physical ailments such as fibromyalgia experience a significant reduction in pain with the addition of therapeutic touch.[2] In a study of Alzheimer's patients, a minimal addition of therapeutic touch, for twenty minutes, reduced both the severity and the frequency of behavioral symptoms of the disease; patients became more present and lucid when they were touched, even for only five minutes at a time.[3]

New evidence shows that even brief touch produces immediate changes in how people react to and process information. For example, students who are touched on their backs or arms by their teachers are twice as likely to participate in class.[4] Human touch from a doctor can significantly strengthen the doctor-patient relationship.[5] In the sports arena, all the high-fiving and body bumping is actually improving athletic performance.[6] As for touching the people we live with, even a brief massage is correlated with decreased depression symptoms and stronger relationships.[7]

Touch wakes up the prefrontal areas of our brain, which control our ability to relax and emote. Holding someone creates a surge of oxytocin, a hormone that helps create a sensation of trust. Even a touch to the shoulder sends a message to the brain that is heard louder than words of support. Touch tells us that someone has our back to share the load, which is one of the primary impetuses for human relationships. I envy Europeans their easy habit of leaning forward and brushing cheeks with almost everyone they meet!

Much of our mistrust of physical affection is learned, and the rigid personal boundary space we establish in response to these lessons often only serves later to prevent our earnest desire to connect. Our discomfort with, and lack of understanding of, our sexuality inadvertently colors our capacity to connect even through something as benign as a hug. I remember listening with both shock and grief as my thirteen-year-old daughter shared how she was warned at school for hugging her boyfriend. "You can't hug for more than two seconds," she was told.

Virginia Satir, who is often referred to as the mother of family therapy, is credited with proposing that we need four hugs a day for survival, eight hugs a day for maintenance, and twelve hugs a day for growth. Her prescription is backed by research that consistently demonstrates that our emotional well-being is deeply impacted by the physical love we experience and that touch and hugging are primary vehicles in the brain's development of basic positive emotions.[8]

As in the mind, so in the body. Recent medical research at the University of North Carolina found that both blood pressure and levels of cortisol, the hormone produced when we're under stress, were significantly lowered (particularly in women) when subjects hugged their partners for at least twenty seconds.[9] Another study that took place in 2013 showed that gently touching infants after a painful medical procedure kept their heart rates steadier.[10] Other studies suggest a strong link between increased hugs and a lower risk of heart disease.[11]

In addition to its clear health benefits, hugging also provides a window into the health of your relationship while also offering an easy way to improve it. "Hugging until relaxed," a therapeutic technique introduced by David Schnarch in *Passionate Marriage*, is a deceptively simple yet transformative practice. Both partners stand on their own two feet and hold each other for at least ten minutes—more if necessary—until both are completely relaxed, first into themselves and then into each other's arms and presence. This holding period is challenging, given that the average hug lasts five seconds. Many of us never really learned to relax in a hug. Learning to relax fully in the arms of someone else, even someone you have been intimate with, requires a new level of trust in yourself. Knowing that you can really open up and not lose yourself in a sustained hug triggers your brain to think differently, creating what Schnarch refers to as a "somatosensory" moment of meeting, which means that we meet each other deeply with our whole bodies. This allows both you and your partner to open up to a deeply intimate space where you can both be held and fully relaxed, which translates into better overall communication and more passionate intimacy. (You'll find more about Schnarch's work in "Further Reading and Resources.")

Opening up to being held is a powerful metaphor, and nowhere is the language of touch more powerful than in your own home. Seemingly small gestures like a kiss goodbye every morning translate into safer driving and increased earnings for the one being kissed. Since learning this, my husband and I have instituted a ritual of holding each other tightly upon returning home each evening, inhaling and grounding each other in our scent and resetting our breathing together. Just a few minutes of coordinating our breathing does wonders for our ability to connect after a long day. It has also seriously reduced the irritability that evenings used to provoke. I have worked to incorporate this practice of holding in my relationships with my children and have seen similar results. Their response to my physical approach tells more than their words ever could about what is happening with them and between us.

When we give it our full attention and bring it to our erotic conversations, touch takes on heightened meaning. We can say more with our hands than we can with our words, and little is misunderstood when the body receives true communication from the hands. Yet inattentive touch, the kind that makes a teenage boy wonder whether fingering "does anything," can also make a body recoil. The pawing and groping that is often associated with teenage sexual discovery doesn't always yield as we age to the subtle and sweeping capacity of touch that the hands hold. Many of us never become really comfortable with our ability to touch even ourselves sexually, and so we never learn how to use our hands to touch others in the many ways we are capable of.

Touching and the sharing of your physical body with your partner are driven by the intention you bring to them. Loving touch is the glue that holds couples together during their most challenging moments, but touch without loving mindfulness can and does undermine real intimacy. As a form of communication, touch is completely clear—and when it is done unfeelingly or with ulterior motives, it is destructive.

Taking our time is everything. Mindful touching is practically prayer, and it is often lost in the crevasse that exists between "hooking up" and making love. Bringing our full attention to the nerve endings meeting between our fingertips and genital tissue causes a fireworks display. If you are not in a mindless hurry to get somewhere else, lingering in this energetically charged exchange for as long as possible can only make the end better.

This is especially true for those among us who struggle with all forms of sexual dysfunction, whether it is premature ejaculation or inability to orgasm. Although they seem to be opposing problems, the answer to both is *slowing down*, focusing on the other and the dance that happens in the container between you. Fingering, touching, feeling the life of your love through your hands is where we begin to experience the harvest of sexual love.

To really touch, we have to bring our full presence to the tips of our fingers. Genital tissue is like none other in the body to touch, and there may be nothing more erotic than spreading oil into the folds and crevices that are as unique as our fingerprints but aglow with far more nerve endings.

》》 Spend a few days consciously aware of how many times you are touched in a day and how many times you reach out to touch someone else. Notice how even the smallest of physical exchanges impacts how you feel in the moment and with the person you touch.

In whatever ways speak to you, try exploring the multitude of ways to touch.

Introducing a variety of different kinds of touch to intimate play is like adding high-octane fuel to your usual moves. There are many erogenous zones on the body beyond the genitalia. Places like the temples, the ear, the nape of the neck, and even the nose carry numerous neuron receptors that will capture your partner's attention and surprise both of you by the stirring they generate.

Don't be afraid to touch yourself while your partner is also caressing or kissing you. That was

never really off limits; we were just self-conscious
teenagers who thought it would be impolite. And
adding different kinds of hand pressure on the
genitals that you are kissing is also fair game.
Experiment with light butterfly fingers or a firm
circular pressure that starts at the base of the penis
and slowly moves upward.

Notice your ability to feel expanding.

Learning to listen—deeply listen—to the world around us is another
ability that we often lose touch with over time. Because we work so
hard to filter out sounds of city noise, like traffic and sirens, we often
lose touch with listening itself. In doing so, we lose a great deal of
texture in our intimate lives. Sound is healing.

We are hardwired to try to make sense of music, and our experience
of it is at once highly complex and also universal. For instance, sad and
happy music evoke consistent emotional responses in babies as young
as nine months old.[12] Our physiology changes when we listen to music.
Dopamine levels peak, for example, and multiple brain regions activate in response to rousing chords or emotional climaxes, producing
feelings of euphoria and even chills.[13] Our favorite songs can give us
the same hit of happiness chocolate can, make us high the way drugs
can, or ignite sexual ecstasy. This isn't that surprising, considering that
our auditory cortex, where vibrations become sound in the brain, also
activates multiple regions associated with emotions, movement, and
memory, which are all fundamental to living inside our sexual selves.

My sexuality has grown up with a very specific playlist. Ever since
I can remember, my lovemaking with my husband has been played
out with a familiar soundtrack, animating our sexual encounter with
its rhythm and bass in the background. It probably began as our way
of covering up anything that might have been overheard by our kids
sleeping down the hall, but slowly and imperceptibly, my dedication
to the artist of the year (or, as my husband would probably argue,
artist of the decade) and the familiar notes of my habitual go-to songs

became a powerful aphrodisiac, both igniting my memory of previous sexual interludes and awakening my sleeping libido.

But it isn't just music that evokes the erotic in us. Sounds of all kinds resonate in the body and enhance the connection to the erotic, especially the sounds that come from within us. I am a little embarrassed to admit that I was nearing my second decade of marriage before I gave up repressing the noises that wanted to erupt from me during sex. While silent urgency has some thrill to it, setting loose the wide range of sounds that our animal sexuality generates is incredibly freeing and erotic. There is something primordial about the sounds sex generates, and whether you are with a new partner or one you have loved for a long time, sounding out in sex heightens everything—your vulnerability, your intimacy, your passion. We growl, purr, grunt, and hiss as well as any other mammal, and maybe better, as our ability to articulate the sounds of love into language waits on the tip of our tongue.

Diving deep into our sexual selves requires a leap—a leap out of our normal day-to-day physical, mental, and emotional boundaries—and a willingness to release our conscious, controlling mind in exchange for the pursuit of passion and pleasure. Attending to the powerful world of sound during lovemaking can help with that leap and can connect you and your partner in new and magical ways. Sound, in its most basic form as noises that we generate, creates resonance between our body and the body nearby. Connecting through sound has the added benefit of turning off our critical minds. It is impossible to simultaneously express a deep *ah* and be thinking about your self-doubts. Primal pleasure takes over and shuts off the ego that can interfere with deep connection. And there is little room for miscommunication when we are forthcoming with the sounds of our true arousal. In fact, there may be no more direct way to tell your partner when they find the magic spot than to let them hear your voice rise an octave. Sound without words invites your partner into the mystery of your arousal and in turn heats up their own arousal.

As you experiment with sounds during lovemaking, keep in mind that your sexy voice is different from your everyday communicating voice.

So be bold, trying out new ranges, from low guttural whispers to high-pitched squeals. Experiment with the tenor of your voice; moving between uncertainty and command carries its own thrill. Paying attention to the layer of sound in your lovemaking not only provides a deeper texture to your pleasure but also clues you in to how clear your communication can be without words. I have also found that sounds surrounding orgasmic pleasure balance the energy vibrating through me and open the way to a deeper release.

Most exciting of all is that freeing your voice can provide a gateway to finding the language to ask in new ways for what you want sexually. Playfully taking on the voice of a ravished submissive or a dominant boor, especially if these are completely out of character in your daily relationship, brings fantasy to life and offers a surprising and passion-inducing twist for even the most familiar of lovers.

Using fantasy voices also encourages the transition that so many struggle with—talking dirty to their partners. I remember well how daring it felt to use the F word when I meant it in the deepest possible way. Although most of us were taught not to swear, using your own sexy lingo makes some of the most forbidden of curse words take on new resonances. Exchanging the sanitary *vagina* and *penis* for slang words that hold forbidden power and meaning feels natural, almost instinctive, and invites you into a whole new level of play.

Expect a certain level of discomfort when you begin moving from guttural sounds and deep purrs into words. One easy way to begin is to describe the sensations of the moment. A purring sound could slip into "I love the feel of your fingers on my…" Encourage your partner to find words, too, by asking questions like "How do you like this motion on your…?"

But as you experiment, keep in mind that different people have different sensual sensitivities, and shared sensation of all types does have to be negotiated. My husband is very sensitive to sound. A door slamming somewhere in the house is enough to make him jump. His interest in and appreciation for a very diverse library of music is something I lack; he can be carried away during a symphony while I am falling asleep. Likewise, during sex, the intensity and range of noises that sometimes erupt from me can be hard for him.

My husband's sensitivity to sound underscores for me the need to acknowledge and make room for the real sensory differences between partners in a relationship. What smells good to you won't always smell as good to your partner. Likewise, what sounds good to you may not please your partner's ears. It's important to keep communicating about what feels good to you both. And while he doesn't ask me to curb my guttural enthusiasm, I try to give my husband warnings of when I am about to explode. This kind of communication is very sexy, bringing a whole new level of engagement to your intimacy.

But maybe the most important thing that we can bring to our most intimate communication is our ability to *listen*. Listening takes time and our full attention. We are not listening when we are already formulating a response. We are not listening when we need to be heard. Truly listening, the way we do when we immerse ourselves in music, happens when we don't just hear the words our partner is saying but also sense the emotion and energy behind the words. Developing our deeper ear for true listening slows down the response that the mind is formulating and allows us to hear the real meaning behind the words being spoken.

Most people struggle to find the words they need to communicate their suffering and pain. And even though I often have felt like I could give them an answer to their struggles without fully hearing them out, what most people really need is the patient silence of a listening ear to come to their own conclusions. Listening is so fundamental to feeling loved that most people cannot tell them apart. Learning to listen better is one of love's most advanced practices and offers the magical space of sensory connection, where the person speaking has the chance to reveal their own learning in the genuine embrace of someone's deep attention and love.

>> Many meditation rituals are steeped in the practice of resonant chanting, which attunes the energy field and body rhythms, connecting us to ourselves and to

the world outside ourselves. The effects of rhythmic sound, breath, and movement during sex are well-known practices in Tantra.

There's one exercise I particularly like because it is simple to learn and demands that both partners commit their full attention to each other. During penetration, it calls for ten shallow strokes followed by one deep stroke, then nine shallow strokes and two deep, and so on, while both partners share breath and sound cues to stay together on "shallow" and "deep" for each stroke. Not only is the practice fully embodying for both partners but also in training your attention so deeply on each other's experience, you share equally in the level of excitement and orgasmic anticipation. It is harder than you think to count all the way down to one shallow stroke and nine deep.

For more information about Tantric practices like this one, see "Further Reading and Resources."

It is odd how we take for granted the most basic of our sensory capacities until life teaches us otherwise. Deterioration of our sight is common to most of us as we age. Although both my parents wore corrective lenses, I boasted perfect vision until suddenly, as I approached fifty, small print became illegible. It was the first real wake-up call for what was coming. Suddenly I started to pay attention to what I could see well and maybe even more attention to what I could no longer see. My attention alone made colors more vivid, gave the subtle textures of fabrics and plants more depth; even the tones of the gray, overcast sky became subtler.

Around this time, I read about a special mom's group for the blind. I tried to imagine what it would be like to never see my child's face light up with a smile or crumple in sadness. The mothers in the article said that because they couldn't *see* their children's emotions, they had to feel for them differently. They trained themselves to listen for different cues, voice intonations, and even energetic fields in the room.

Many of us who have vision never take the time to really see *what* or, more tragically, *who* is in front of us. Taking our eyesight for granted, we frequently get blinded by the insistence that we can look at two, three, four, or more things simultaneously, kidding ourselves that we can take it all in. We can't and don't, and our perceptions are compromised when we don't take the time to singularly focus on any single topic or person. This is especially true when it comes to discerning meaning on someone's face. When we accelerate our visual stimulus to digital levels, we lose the ability to gaze deeply into someone's eyes for the information they can't put into words. We only see what we are prepared to comprehend, which explains why we so often walk away from our closest interpersonal encounters feeling invisible.

Like listening deeply, seeing deeply requires our full attention, so that our heart can engage to both inform and filter our vision. This deeper seeing is a kind of curious and compassionate witnessing that feels like an embrace. We are literally holding someone in our regard, which heals both the person being seen and the person looking. This focused attention speaks love, and it rewards us with a fresh perspective on issues that keep us apart. We learn in this authentic seeing that we can change our situation and improve our intimate connection just by the way we choose to look at it. Trusting the emotional intelligence that comes with our full attention is often all we need to see our relationship with new eyes.

Learning to see what is right in front of us requires a slowing down of the mental chatter. Instead of the fast processing speed we apply to most everything else, we pause, we breathe, and we focus. Think to yourself, as you look at your lover's hand chopping vegetables or look into the eyes of your beloved pet, "What if this were the last time I witnessed this?" Now look again. Everything slows down to its true time. Truly seeing is bearing witness, and it brings reverence to every act—especially the sexual ones, as we give up all our preconceived notions of beauty in favor of the magnificence of living in this body, entangled with erotic connection to another body. Making love with our eyes open to the world around us softens the harshest edges and allows us to witness the moments in between the perpetual departure, which is this life.

>> Begin this training in the daily moments of waking, eating, and living side by side. Even for only five seconds, look up and see the person speaking to you across the kitchen counter. Look up and hold your partner's gaze when they share their concerns about the car or the kids. The practice of training your eyes on the ones you love, at first for five seconds and extending that to thirty, will teach you the truth of finding eternity in a minute. It will also prepare you for the simplest yet most extraordinary shift you can make in your physical lovemaking. The vast majority of couples make love in the dark, eyes shut. Bringing light, cracking your eyes open to witness the person above or below you while you share the most intimate poses, will surprise, bewilder, and connect you like nothing else.

My sensory life came alive through my nose. As I mentioned, a chance purchase of a bottle of love oil set me on a course that helped me cultivate a deep appreciation for scent. Back when I had just begun to investigate the distinct qualities of different scents and how their combinations created entirely new experiences, I became increasingly curious about why and how scent so powerfully impacts not only our immediate erotic experience but also memory itself. Lewis Thomas, a physician and an engaging essayist, wrote, "The act of smelling something, anything, is remarkably like the act of thinking itself. Immediately, at the very moment of perception, you can feel the mind going to work, sending the odor around from place to place, setting off complex repertoires throughout the brain, polling one center after another for signs of recognition, old memories, connections."[14]

Our sense of smell is our most primal way of knowing our world and has a potent influence on memory, emotion, and behavior. Unlike visual and auditory information—signals detected by our eyes and ears—scent information bypasses the thalamus, a sort of sensory way station, and goes directly to the olfactory cortex for instant processing.[15] Like other mammals, we also depend on scent to discern sexual compatibility, and the mechanism for doing so is built into the limbic brain, one of the most primal structures of our brains. A first kiss is also a first opportunity to imperceptibly but without question know if this other person could be our match. Each of us has a genetic scent makeup that is as unique as our fingerprint. In fact, our sense of smell and what attracts or repels us to others is blueprinted in the part of our immunological gene structure called the major histocompatibility complex (MHC).[16]

What's more, when it comes to reproduction, the healthiest progeny comes from two individuals whose MHC is most distinct and different from each other; this ensures that any offspring has the widest range of immune function and therefore is the most disease-resistant.[17] This makes perfect evolutionary sense—and it also profoundly affects the whole courting process, as well as the likelihood of making your love sustainable. MHC compatibility is a predictor not only of bearing healthy offspring but also of relationship longevity and the frequency of infidelity.[18]

Even more remarkable than this biological basis of scent compatibility between partners is the new recognition that our ability to smell is intimately entwined with our ability to feel. Recent research on people who suffer anosmia (scent blindness) shows that they are more likely to become depressed, as well as unable to feel a wide range of emotions.[19] Research shows that we find things both more beautiful and memorable when they are combined with a pleasant scent.[20] We know this intuitively when we are hungry; almost any food looks more appetizing when accompanied by an attractive smell. Marketers use this to their advantage; casinos, hotels, large shopping malls, and theme parks all routinely pipe in pleasant scents, which have positive effects on everything from how long people stay to how much money they spend. Other studies have demonstrated that both women and men rank photos of the opposite sex higher when they view them while smelling a pleasant odor as opposed to an unpleasant or a neutral odor.[21]

What attracts us or repels us about another person's scent is not only as unique as we are but also not negotiable. There is no cure for scent incompatibility, while scent compatibility can drive us wild with desire. (Napoleon was notorious for requesting that his wife, Josephine, not wash for a week before he came home.) Even the use of heavily scented colognes or perfumes will not mask scent incompatibility for long. We have neural pathways deep in our brains that are normally reserved for making the distinction between fearsome and familiar stimuli, but they can also detect scent compatibility. This is the way nature protects us from mating with people who are too biologically similar to us. As with other mammals, our sense of smell has evolved for our survival. Covering up your own natural odor may actually interfere with your ability to be found (or smelled by) your true mate.

These facts belie the scant attention that we often give to our olfactory sense. In part, this is because we have so little language for scent. Not uncommonly, scent language is often limited to "it smells like . . ." and our recognition of scents often only gets as far as broad categories, pleasant and unpleasant. But like all our other senses, the olfactory is developmental, which means that through attention and practice, we can expand our ability to both smell and identify scents. It is a worthwhile effort, as new research reveals how the complex ways we process olfactory stimuli color everything, from how we feel, to what we see and hear, to what we remember.[22]

Expanding the language of your nose by paying more attention to the scents surrounding you is both mind-expanding and memory building, because it brings you fully into the present moment. Scent, more than any of our other senses, is processed alongside the same pathways that code our emotions and memories. In other words, recognizing smells enriches our experience in the moment and enhances our ability to remember it afterward. It is no accident that our arousal mechanism is equally influenced by this process. Waking up to scent and employing it strategically with intimate partners can be a game changer for romance. So take this message to heart, and as you breathe, inhale deeply and build your vocabulary and experience of scent, especially with the people you love most.

>> Here are the instructions that I have offered people for the use of scented aphrodisiac oil, which I call "love oil" (see the appendix). Love oils can be used with any scented oil that the two of you love. Rub the oil into all the places you want your lover to kiss you. Be exotic. Start at your feet—say maybe the curve of the ankle—and work up from there. Let him sniff his way up your body. To make it even more tantalizing, make it an inhale-only tour. No mouth kissing, just inhaling you, or as my husband likes to say, "Smoking you."

As the excitement builds, find your way back to the wrist. Have your lover find your pulse with their lips. Keep your eyes open, and watch them holding your life on their lips, watching you watch them. Then find your lover with your own lips, as I know you must, and make that first kiss as slow and luxurious as you can. Just a hint of tongue, of what is to come.

Whatever your preference, know that our olfactory system is our primary sense when it comes to attraction. Throughout history, our sense of smell has been crucial to the art of mating. Use it to your advantage. Trust your sense of smell to excite you, and indulge in whatever scents turn you on.

Our sense of taste both relies on and heightens many of our other senses. All of our favorite foods, as well as those we find repelling, make their

>> Do an experiment next time you are searching for the desire to have sex: instead of thinking about sex, wake up your senses.

Think about your next sexual encounter as a gourmet meal of many courses and flavors. Remember the last fabulous multicourse meal you had—hors d'oeuvres, salad, coffee, fruit, dessert. Remember the flavors, the conversation, the lingering touches.

Now apply that same attention to your partner. Use a little love oil to highlight your own pheromones and your awareness of the scent chemistry between you and your partner. The arousal mechanism stirs—and so does your partner's body—as the oil glides to the curves and valleys of the body. Why hurry to the main course when there is so much to savor along the way?

Adding another scent as a second step extends the pleasure, introducing a whole new synergy of scent and flavor when we are kissing our most sensitive tissues. Flooded with sensuality, we feel the pressure lighten and the pleasure turn on.

This is the moment when a penetration aid, like personal lubricant, can really do its job, adding the old familiar slip to the deepest communion we can manifest.

Hurrying to the main course is anticlimactic at best, painful at worst. Take time to explore what it means to feel sensuous.

One of my favorite movie scenes comes from the 1987 Wim Wenders film *Wings of Desire*. Peter Falk is speaking to an angel he senses next to him. He is bubbling with gratitude about the joy of living in a body, the deep satisfaction of physical human experience, found in an act as small and often unnoticed as warming one's hands on a cold winter night with a steaming cup of coffee. He lingers over the strong aroma cutting the night air and the warmth of his breath puffing over the cup. He laughs at the feeling of tingling heat coming back into his numb fingers. I remember this scene each and every time I catch myself taking this bodily experience for granted.

When it comes to living in a body and experiencing the world through our remarkable five senses, attention and appreciation are one and the same. Our attention is the rare and purest form of gratitude that happens when we stop and use our senses fully, allowing our heart and higher mind to bask in the wonder and mystery of our human bodies. Poet Mary Oliver wrote, "This is the first, wildest, and wisest thing I know: that the soul exists, and that it is built entirely out of attentiveness."[24]

Experiencing this amazing world through our miraculous physical body is nothing if not a sensory feast. In fact, it is impossible not to experience this generous attending to even the smallest of details without being overcome by our basic capacity to feel, smell, and taste. Just imagine for a moment losing any one of those senses. Imagine that you might never again smell the sweet freshness of early morning or awaken to the sensation of a soft pillow meeting your head. This is where the privilege of living inside of a body becomes so tender—when we realize how fleeting and perfect so many of our small visceral moments really are. Even the brilliant color bursts of the trees on their way to dormancy shake me wide awake these days. Imagine a day without color, and then look around.

7

FANTASY

Within you is all of the erotic fuel you will ever need to have passionate sex with the same person for the rest of your life. You can access this fuel any time by tapping its deep source: your inner fantasy life. The fantasy life I am referring to is not to be confused with the daydreaming thoughts about your next vacation or winning the lottery. What I'm referring to are your most deeply arousing intimate fantasies—fantasies that are so intrinsic to the essence of your being that you may not even be consciously aware of them.

My goal in this chapter is not to tell you what fantasies you should be having—only you can find that out. And I am not going to tell you how to have fantasies, or what your fantasies mean, or whether you should play out your fantasies with your partner. What I want to share with you is more basic than any of that, but in many ways more challenging: I want to show you that the key to unlocking your never-ending sexual fuel is to become fully aware of and a true *witness* to your own fantasies.

As you open to consciously witnessing your fantasies, you begin to return to the uninhibited sexuality that you first felt in adolescence, the time when many of us were also learning, from family and society, to feel ashamed of our sexual urges. The earliest and usually most potent emotional wounds we incur are the stuff that our subconscious mind is working to heal as our erotic selves emerge. The fantasies that are most sexually charged can help us to reinterpret the painful parts of our past and turn them into something pleasurable. Just by starting to acknowledge the fantasies that you have carried with you over the years, you heal those old wounds and open up that inexhaustible reserve of fuel for a passionate intimate life.

Like most of the healing work I have been describing in this book, reclaiming our fantasies for erotic fuel isn't something we just do once and then we're set for life. For me, as for most people, it takes a continuous effort to consciously open up to my fantasy life and let it lead me into the deepest spaces of arousal. Life has a way of challenging everything we think we know, demonstrating over and over that the learning is never really done. Not that long ago, I found myself in a situation that taught me yet again just how powerful fantasies can be when instead of trying to act them out, we learn to use them like an ignition switch for our own private reserves of erotic energy.

It all started with a leak under my refrigerator. Soon it became clear that the entire wood floor needed replacing. After my contractor arrived, it was agreed that the old cabinets would look even worse than they already did next to a new floor, so now I had a job in the kitchen rehab project. Before long, the kitchen was gutted, and I was working alongside my contractor sanding and refinishing.

What makes guys who can fix things so sexy? Contractors have always been one of my weaknesses; I can't seem to help falling for guys with power tools. And I know I am not alone in my contractor fantasies: there are entire erotic books and porn series dedicated to the theme. At the time, the situation felt charged and sexual, but looking back, I don't know if my contractor had any idea about the sexual energy that working alongside him evoked in me. As he showed me the tricks of cleaning out a belt sander or set up sawhorse workstations for me, our time together resonated with small gestures of flirtation that made me laugh out loud at myself through the sawdust. But even though I think I stayed outwardly cool about it, the thrill of getting so close to my contractor fantasy caught me off guard. Through the fog of my menopausal hot flashes, something girly and unexpected bubbled up in me as we weighed the merits of gloss or satin. I couldn't remember the last time I felt my libido rising in the presence of a younger man.

And I remembered again how much sexual energy is tied up in small flirtatious exchanges like these. Even a tiny dose of this kind of attentive attraction feels like a happy drug. I felt like I was sipping from the proverbial fountain of youth.

It was all in my mind, of course. And yet these initial surprising and sweet feelings quickly became riddled with guilt and confusion as I struggled with that question that confronts so many of us when real life brings us so close to our fantasies: what am I supposed to *do* with this? I knew enough not to act on such a fantasy and risk my family and the profoundly remarkable physical intimacy I share with my husband, yet I also sensed that I shouldn't turn away from this exciting sexual energy arising in me, as if my fantasy life were a threat. That energy felt urgent, like something I had to act on right away or miss out on for the rest of my life. And even though I had already worked hard to develop an open and comfortable relationship with my internal fantasy life, I was unprepared for how this real-life fantasy expanded all the ways I felt lonely and neglected in my marriage.

I had to take a deep breath and remind myself of what I already knew: the best thing to do with this erotic energy of fantasy is not to act on it, but to witness it and bring it into my real-life relationship. When we deny our fantasies or mistake them for reality, they can do incredible damage to our erotic lives. But when we fully acknowledge and witness them, these fantasies can heal the very weaknesses they expose in our relationships.

I'll give another example—one that happened before I learned to witness my fantasies. Years before I met that contractor, when I first started Good Clean Love, I found myself in a similar situation. Back then, I had not yet recognized all the ways that acting out a fantasy can be dangerous and damaging to my intimate relationship or, even worse, the ways it could confuse my own erotic urges.

Peter, as we'll call him, was a charismatic leader in the green business community. Something about his energy and his smile stirred something deep in my erotic soul and ignited my arousal mechanism in a way I couldn't remember it being ignited before. Just a single kiss turned my world upside down, and a fantasy life (over which I had little control at the time) grabbed me by my heels and filled me with the addictive anticipation of seeing him again. For a while we stayed connected, sending emails charged with that magical elixir that had been sparked by an unforgettable kiss.

It didn't take long for my husband to sense something and for me to notice how impossible it was becoming for me to stay present in my marriage. Despite the kiss and the emails, it was a fantasy—just thoughts passing through my mind without much substance—but I felt like I had to hide something. I didn't yet understand that what was most precious about the fantasy, and even the kiss with Peter, was that it fueled my own libido, and that I could use that fuel to make my sex life with my husband not just good, but incredible. As time went on, my preoccupation with Peter distracted me from the intimate life right in front of me. Peter became my mental escape hatch every time things were challenging with my husband. I was lucky I realized, before it did too much damage, what a player Peter was and that he really cared nothing for me or my life.

There was still a lot that I didn't understand about accessing the power of fantasy when I met Peter. I had yet to open up to the erotically charged fantasy playground living in my own mind, so it was easy for me, as it is for so many people, to mistake the thoughts inspired by random sexually charged meetings for something I had to act on for them to have any value. We tend not to value the spark of a sexual encounter if we don't act on it, believing that acting on it makes it real, valuable. Yet this distinction is *critical* when it comes to unlocking the power of fantasy: the spark is actually more valuable, not less, if we refrain from acting on it and instead use its energy to fuel our erotic life—not only because our internal fantasy playground offers so much opportunity for erotic awakening and potential healing but also because it doesn't carry nearly the same risk as engaging with real-life scenarios that often end up leaving us in a heap of disappointment and pain.

Perhaps one of the best analogies for understanding this critical aspect of fantasy is the act of masturbation. Masturbation is the cornerstone of our sexual identity; and while often it is something we do privately, it helps us practice for partnered sex, familiarizing us with the kind of intimate touch we prefer and teaching us how to modulate our reaction time so that we can synchronize with our partner. Also, the more comfortable we become with masturbation, the more powerful an ally it can be during sex with our partners. Masturbation is also something we can do during partnered sex. It can be an incredibly sexy and intimately bonding experience to touch yourself in front of your partner and to watch while your partner does the same. It can also be instructive, opening a space for dialogue about how you and your partner might like to be touched by each other. As an aid to intimacy, masturbation parallels how fantasy works: the more comfortable we become with our own fantasies, the more they can fuel our partnered experiences.

If masturbation helps us become familiar with our body's pleasure responses, fantasies provide the same insight into our erotic mind. As we become more comfortable with our fantasies and learn what really turns us on, we gain a sense of mastery over our own capacity for arousal. Bringing this increased confidence into sex with a partner, we can effortlessly tap into our most erotic fantasies—either silently, in our own mind, or by sharing them aloud. Either way, when engaged with consciously, fantasies add a dimension to sex that makes the experience both more visceral and, perhaps paradoxically, more real, because our fantasies are the most unique expressions of our own authentic sexuality—our sexual thumbprint, if you will.

However, moderation is important. Too much masturbation and likewise an obsession with fantasy life can physically numb us to another's touch or accustom us to a narrow range of sexual experiences. Both masturbation and fantasy can be aids to intimacy when practiced in moderation, but hinder us when we rely on them too much.

Whether we're working alongside a sexy contractor, regularly encountering a handsome coworker by the water cooler, or running into an old flame by chance, it is not unusual to find ourselves in erotically charged situations that quickly evolve into fantasy. Arguably, these are some of the most titillating situations we encounter, and they hold a great deal of fuel for our erotic fire—and consequently for our relationships—when we recognize their erotic charge but don't act on that charge with the person who happened to trigger it. When that contractor pulled up to my house in his Chevy, things could have unfolded very differently than they did. Had I not already become so comfortable with my interior sexual fantasies, I know it would have been easy for me to confuse the rush of sexual energy that arises during brief fantasies with the far greater pleasure that comes from doing the work to stay loving in my own relationship—work that is fueled by a rich private fantasy life.

>> Try to remember the last time you were faced with an erotically charged sexual encounter that arose in the course of your daily life. Write down some of the feelings that emerged for you, both positive and negative.

Next, close your eyes and imagine that experience as though it were a dream. Do any of your feelings change? What is the most arousing part of the encounter in your dream? Is this different than what turned you on in real life?

Notice this change of perspective from the dream space to three-dimensional reality. Many people find that the dream arousal leads them to understand something more elusive about the situation. Dare to dig deeper.

Unlocking the power of fantasy begins with *witnessing* our fantasies—simply seeing, with clear, nonjudging eyes, what really turns us on. Make no mistake: unlocking the door to our private fantasy world isn't easy. One of my most vivid memories from my early twenties shows how deeply disturbing our own erotic impulses can be and just how difficult it can be to witness our arousal without judgment.

I was living in Minneapolis with my husband, and one day I found myself at the Como Park Zoo, probably the last zoo in the country to keep huge animals in small cages that visitors could walk right up to. As I turned the corner, I heard the roar of a lion before I fully understood what was happening. There, not more than ten feet away, were two huge lions copulating ferociously. The roars were deafening (as you might expect from a lion!).

I was captivated. Even though I was by myself, I remember feeling both sexually excited and ashamed. For the few minutes that it lasted, I couldn't take my eyes off their encounter. I was stunned by the power of the act, but even more so by my own response. Immediately the sexual police in my head started their interrogation: why was I aroused watching lions have sex? Back then, for me, as for most people, shame was never far from my arousal mechanism.

The sex between the lions stayed with me for years. I was never quite able to forget it and never really sure why I was so captivated by their sex—or why shame was always such a close companion to my arousal.

Then, in my early days as a loveologist, I came across a research study conducted by Meredith Chivers and had the good luck of getting an interview with her.[1] Her research focused on the differences in arousal response between genders, comparing different kinds of stimuli. The women in the study were hooked up to a plethysmograph (which measures vaginal blood flow and lubrication) and shown a variety of porn clips—sex between men and women, women and women, men and men, and a pair of bonobos. The results of the women's trial (which included both straight and lesbian women) were surprising: all the women were aroused by all of the different sexual acts, including the copulating apes. Chivers performed the same trial with both gay and straight men, who responded in more expected patterns: straight men's arousal soared when women were on screen and sagged when men were on screen. Gay men had the opposite response. Neither male group responded at all to the apes.

The interesting conclusion was that women become aroused when they witness sex—any kind of sex. Unfortunately, the results of Chivers's study were misunderstood and quickly skewed in the media. Articles began coming out claiming a new study had shown that women really want sex all the time, even when they say no. There was a backlash and the predictable media circus. But the original study gave rise to a widespread misunderstanding of sexuality, particularly the role of fantasy and imagination in arousal. What wasn't being fully understood, or what was perhaps being willfully overlooked, is that while witnessing something can arouse women, this arousal does not necessarily indicate a desire to participate in or enact what has turned them on. The female response to the clips of copulating apes makes this obvious, as did my experience with the lions. As captivating and erotic as watching them was, I never entertained the idea of participating. In fact, my arousal response depended on my keeping a safe distance, being an observer, separated from the act by a set of strong iron bars. My arousal came from witnessing an experience and then witnessing what my mind did with that experience, which is how fantasies form and live in us.

>> You can most easily learn to witness your fantasy life during masturbation practice. If you have no idea what is lurking inside, try reading a range of erotica (see "Further Reading and Resources" for source material) or watching compelling story-based pornography. For many people, the most challenging part of witnessing their fantasies is not shying away from their "politically incorrect" tone, which fantasies often have. Giving yourself permission to explore this space is the crucial step to opening the door. Remember that your fantasies are private; you don't have to share them with anyone else.

Just as we are each aroused by different kinds and intensities of touch, we each have a powerful inner erotic landscape that reveals itself to us through fantasies, whether we are willing to witness them or not. Many people, as I did for years, spend a lot of energy turning away from their fantasies because they lie so shockingly outside the ways we know ourselves, or because we believe that knowing them will somehow force us to fulfill them, or because we confuse the real-life incidents and the fantasies that ensue as proof that fantasy cannot lead to anything good. For many people, the internal landscape of fantasy is a Pandora's box—better left alone, unopened and unexplored.

I remember how hard I worked to suppress my sexual fantasies in the early years of my marriage. Some of my most vivid memories of sex with my husband during that time are of the many techniques I developed to shut down my sexual memories and all of the bizarre, politically incorrect images and story lines that haunted my libido. The times I would catch glimpses of my fantasies of forced pleasure between inappropriate partners both turned me on and terrified me. Where did these fantasies come from? Was I a victim of some long forgotten abuse? I felt afraid and trapped by these sexual fantasies that came unbidden. I was plagued with questions of my own normality. How could I have come up with this kind of fantasy material? I couldn't talk about it with anyone. Over time, I learned to shut myself off, which took so much attention I found it hard to focus on what I was feeling. Our sex life became a series of moves we knew by rote, and it was brief and lifeless.

It wasn't until the real honeymoon some fifteen years into my marriage, after my husband gave me lingerie for my birthday, that I finally had the courage to take off my fantasy blinders. I was inspired by the collective courage it took for us to find each other again so passionately. It made me bold and allowed me to let my curiosity reign. Although many of the intense images I had glimpsed of inappropriate partners having forced sexual pleasure were still racing around in my mind, I was able finally to let them play freely before my eyes. It was rocket fuel. It was in this way that I learned that turning away from my fantasy life was tantamount to a death sentence for my libido—and I wasn't willing to go back there.

Again, the work of acknowledging our fantasies and bringing them to light is not easy. For most of us, the most troubled relationship we have is not with our partners or children or coworkers; it's with our erotic selves. Most everyone who dives into this erotically charged inner landscape shares questions about where they come from, how our fantasies evolve, and why they turn us on. That nagging question that comes up so frequently about our erotic selves—Is this normal?—peaks when it comes to our fantasy lives. By definition, the content of our fantasies can be disturbing; they usually aren't politically correct or socially appropriate. But fantasies are as persistent as they are strange, and try as we might to block them out, they are always lurking somewhere close behind our arousal mechanism, insisting on being witnessed.

When I finally began to realize how much energy I was using to suppress my fantasies, I became curious about what I had been so afraid to look at. I was stunned and ashamed at the fantasy life that emerged from me. This is where my sexual experience with my husband became truly passionate and surprising, but also a little scary. The fantasies I began letting myself see felt deeply inappropriate, involving being a child or in some other submissive role and being forced into all kinds of sexual acts and even into pleasure itself. These fantasies came unbidden to my mind and were so vivid that for a brief time I wondered if something awful had happened to me as a child and I was only now remembering it. In the end, I came to know that these disturbing yet alluring images were not my memories but rather fabrications of my subconscious mind. But this was not that comforting, because soon I began to worry that something was wrong with me, that these thoughts must be evidence of my own sexual deviance.

My husband is a psychiatrist, but there was no way I could bring myself to tell him about the scenarios playing out in my mind while we had sex. A few times I tried to tell him, but I literally could not get the words out. So I kept them to myself. And while I reveled in how remarkably charged and intense our sex life became, I was also ashamed that my fantasy life was fueled by imagery and story lines too disturbingly taboo to ever share with anyone. It felt like a bizarre double life I was leading. On the one hand, my ability to expand my sexual boundaries through fantasy exploded the ways in which I could experiment with types of sex I had never considered before, and on the other, I was sure I must be some kind of sexual deviant.

Confused and uncertain, I began searching for material that might help me make sense of what was going on. I turned to reading erotica, which both fueled my fantasies and shocked me even more: a *lot* of the books that I read were even more disturbing than my own fantasies. I couldn't imagine writing these stories and putting my name on them. (I didn't realize at first that most erotica writers use pen names.) Reading tales of sexual domination and submission, which were the most riveting for me, added fuel to my fire and also brought me solace, because if I was deviant, then at least I wasn't alone. And it reaffirmed for me that there is a chasm between fantasizing about something in my mind and attempting to enact that content in real time, whether it is some form of consensual rape, domination until it hurts, or forced pleasure in sex work, to name just a few common themes. I knew that enacting my fantasies would be horrifying, whether pleasure was had or not.

Around this time, the runaway bestseller *Fifty Shades of Grey* was reaching the height of its popularity. In case you haven't read it, the story is about a young, beautiful virgin who doesn't recognize her own beauty and a deeply troubled young man who channels his childhood pain and extreme wealth into a fringe sexual lifestyle that verges on violence. The plot twists and turns around submission and dominance, one of the oldest and most common fantasy themes in human history. That this story shifted the sexual landscape of our culture and captivated the attention of millions of readers reveals the singular most significant truth of our collective human sex drive: our access to our fantasies is where our sexual motor revs up or languishes.

One of the most popular themes for many of us as we start to interact with our fantasies involves the act of submission and its corollary, domination. *Fifty Shades of Grey* taps this deep nerve in our collective sexual subconscious. There is something deeply forbidden at the heart of the strange yet compelling relationship between pleasure and submission. What is it about this kind of sexual fantasy that simultaneously revolts and utterly captivates us? The young female virgin consents to a practice of sexuality that engulfs her. She cannot turn away from the danger; she is helpless as she is swept up in the enormity of her previously unknown sexual urges. This notion is at the core of fantasy life—the idea of being so passionately swept up in the sex that we lose control, and as we do, we no longer have to be responsible for our sexual desire. We flip through pages as she submits, has orgasms on command, and endures profound pain. Yet even as her fear melts into unanticipated pleasure, she remains the codependent submissive. Rather than exploring the power of her own desire, the will of her own pleasure, she continues to submit to her dominating and cruel lover.

Fifty Shades of Grey captures the heart of many sexual fantasies: the longing to submit to the intense sexual energy that we all sense at our core and to be absolved, through our submission, of all responsibility for our own desires. In this way, our own desires become forbidden to us. And in a culture where desire is forbidden, where we long to escape from our responsibility for our "forbidden" desires, it's no surprise that there is ongoing confusion over sexual consent. College campuses struggle now to define and teach young adults what is true consent. Many times, our sexuality is a jumble of raw confusion that mistakes consent and right, refusal and wrong, in a myriad of circumstances that easily slip beyond our control. How many of us cannot access our ability to experience pleasure unless it is somehow forbidden? *Fifty Shades of Grey* has so far been translated into fifty-two languages and sold more than 100 million copies worldwide.[2] Ironically, even as we sacrifice a connection with our own fantasies and desires, our appetite for stories of someone else's fantasies increases until it feels insatiable.

Reading erotica expanded my fantasy life to a degree: it reassured me that I was within the range of normal when it comes to having wild fantasies. Yet it didn't really answer my nagging questions about my own fantasies. Why was I so drawn to these particular relationships and story lines? Why, when I entered into the depth of my sexuality with my husband, did my mind consistently go to *these* places?

During the time when I was searching for material to help me make sense of my fantasy life, I was still doing my radio show, and one week I was fortunate enough to get an interview with Stanley Siegel. He was just launching his book *Your Brain on Sex*. This was the moment when the light came on about our sexual fantasies. I still palpably remember my conversation with Stanley and the wonder and relief I felt as he explained how our subconscious minds form sexual fantasies in an attempt to heal the pain and trauma from our childhood by eroticizing the residue of unresolved feelings these experiences imprint on us. This subconscious mechanism begins as we enter puberty and the mind tries to bring pleasure to what has been persistently painful. The pain of isolation or abandonment can be remedied through a wide range of sexual fantasies, which is what makes each person's erotic self so unique. Siegel's thesis is that our sexuality becomes a place of deep healing when we can acknowledge our unresolved childhood feelings and learn to connect to the fantasies that our subconscious minds create as a means of healing.

One point that Stanley reiterated during our interview, I think for my own comfort, is that our fantasy life is not formed through conscious decision or choice; rather, it is formed deep in our subconscious, out of our awareness, which in fundamental ways lets us off the hook. Not realizing this, many people feel a lot of shame and fear about their fantasy life. Collectively we all share in some degree of shame and discomfort with our erotic selves, and consequently it is not uncommon for many of us to entirely repress the strong fantasies that are meant to fuel our arousal and desire.

This repression represents a tragic loss of who we are. Coming to appreciate our sexual fantasies in the context of our whole life experience provides a window into the deepest levels of healing in our psyche. Our sexuality, and the erotic soul that embodies it, is an expression of our most complex human needs, including the remarkable healing drive to experience pleasure. It is impossible to escape childhood without suffering some form of emotional wounding and unresolved conflict. It actually makes a lot of sense that our subconscious, which is always at work to heal us, would, as we mature into our sexuality in early adolescence, eroticize our pain through fantasies that transform our painful past into a pleasurable experience. (You can read more about Stanley's book in "Further Reading and Resources.")

Inspired by Stanley's work, for a time I was determined to find the link between my persistent fantasies and the issues that might have started them. I thought that this was the most urgent work, the work that had to be done before I could be sexually healthy and free. But as time passed, just this understanding—that my fantasies were what were fueling my sex life—was enough to give me the sexual health and freedom I was seeking. I began to deeply appreciate the gift that these fantasies offered up without necessarily having to explore the deepest recesses of my past. In fact, having the courage to simply look at and experience my fantasy life was in its own way therapeutic: it defused some of my old emotional baggage and offered me a bridge by which to access not only my powerfully erotic identity but also, and even more profoundly, a window into my deepest psyche.

Our erotic selves and our sexual needs are secondary only to our other primary needs of eating, drinking, and sleeping. Witnessed from this perspective, our fantasy lives are actually vital to our lives. They provide us the most profound view of our subconscious drive toward healing and experiencing pleasure. To the degree that we suppress the fantasies that live deep in us, we lose not only our access to deep plea- sure but also the wealth of information that these fantasies hold for our own healing. When we work with our fantasies, we are engaging with something fundamental in ourselves, something in the deepest layer of who we are as human beings.

Still, the power that our sexuality exerts in our lives is often misun- derstood and shadowed with shame. Arguably, it is the unspoken and invisible parts of us that dominate our thinking. Even when we believe we are not making decisions based on our sexual needs, we realize later that, in fact, we are. How else can we explain the frequency of poor judgment and inappropriate, hurtful sexual actions that we see at all levels of our society? From our political system to the damage in our families to the vast numbers of sexual slaves around the world, I firmly believe that these are fueled by the covert forces of our unacknowl- edged sexuality. As long as we relate to our sexuality only as a part of ourselves to be controlled and silenced, it will remain the root of our fears about ourselves, our fantasy lives, and about others. As long as we misinterpret our erotic urges and fantasies as base and primitive instincts that have to be contained, our sexual fantasies and even desire itself will be walled off and our sex lives deadened.

Acknowledging and creating a relationship with the barrier of fear that perpetuates both our distance from and misunderstanding of our erotic selves begins with learning to engage with our fantasies. As I mentioned earlier in this chapter, the first step is to be willing to look at and identify your persistent fantasies. As a way of deepening your witnessing, you might consider where these fantasies come from, where in your past they originate. But keep in mind that just as it isn't necessary or desirable to act out our fantasies, it isn't always necessary to go digging for their sources. You can experience great sexual freedom just by witnessing your fantasies without judgment. That means not adding any labels, like "too wild" or "too tame" or "not kinky enough." There's a vast range of what's "normal" when it comes to our fantasy life, just as there is when it comes to sex.

Personally, I have found that connecting my fantasies with my early life experiences gives me a better sense of how my mind works to make sense of and heal my most painful, wounded places. When I began to understand my fantasies in the context of my subconscious and my childhood traumas, the connections to my childhood feelings of being out of control and threatened by authority figures with physical punishment made sense of my submissive fantasies. I wondered, and then worried, whether making the connection to my emotional wounds would make the fantasies go away. However, I've found that what has gone away is the *shame* I felt about my fantasy life. My fantasy life itself, far from vanishing, has evolved. As I began to consistently witness and accept my fantasies, I became bolder in the kinds of erotica I was reading and seeing. As a result, different kinds of fantasies emerged that made my sex life even more intense and exciting.

As I've learned and relearned countless times, most recently with the contractor described at the beginning of this chapter, the real power of fantasy comes from witnessing. But are there contexts in which enacting our fantasies can take us even further? Undeniably, the space between witnessing and enacting is huge, and enacting our fantasies in 3D can have real, lasting consequences for us and our relationships. There are many avenues, from getting involved in sex work to frequenting dungeons, by which to explore the full expression of just about any fantasy imaginable. Making a decision to experience our fantasies in the real world changes life in ways both big and small. For some, there is an amazing surge of courage that comes with finally living out a long-hidden fantasy, but for plenty of others, living out fantasies hurts the people involved in all sorts of unexpected ways. At the very least, if you do choose to bring your fantasies to life, remember that it's even more important to practice safe dating and sex!

Because I have experienced the amazing power of fantasy as a private source of rocket fuel for my erotic self, I believe that this is an extremely powerful place to begin with empowering your erotic experience. I would even venture that for most people, bringing our internal fantasies to life is anticlimactic; just having them is enough to keep you revved up for a long time. As soon as we begin to act them out, they lose a great deal of their power; the spark of fantasy goes out very quickly, leaving us feeling exposed.

It isn't as if I have never considered bringing my fantasies into the real world. For example, I have sometimes fantasized about bringing into our bedroom a third woman whom only I could direct. Even though the idea is pretty exciting, when I consider the consequences and how many unknowns there are, I do not come close to acting on this. Although I have shared this fantasy with my husband, we both acknowledge that we don't really know how it would feel for us to have someone else present and how it would impact what would happen for us afterward. We agree that witnessing our fantasies gives us plenty of fuel. It works powerfully enough that I can just leave this one in my head.

When my fantasies become dangerous or frightening, I still find myself coming back to this place of witness. Sometimes, if the imagery or sensation gets too intense or brings me too deeply in touch with the terror that the real experience might evoke, I change the channel. But I also have gained an ever-deepening compassion for sexual-abuse survivors and increasingly an ability to act in the world to stop the rampant levels of pain that ignorant sexuality creates. Knowing our own risk tolerance for how deeply we can interact with our fantasies is personal, and it takes practice. Mature adult relationships recognize that there will always be a long-term impact that comes from moving private fantasy into waking reality, and that this should not be easily dismissed by the attitude that "I'm just experimenting." My advice is to go slow. Be cautious and thoughtful with this precious combustible energy. Begin by wanting to witness what is happening inside, and let it play out slowly, if at all, in the world.

Only on very rare occasions do I articulate my fantasies to my husband. Much more often, I have allowed the animal girl that I am in my fantasies to express herself with sounds—so even when my husband doesn't know the content of my fantasies, he definitely gets the gist. Really, there is so much rich and juicy libido waiting to be tapped inside of us. All it takes is the willingness to witness our fantasies, to completely see them without judgment or shame.

8

ATTENTION

As a writer on the topic of pleasure, I have often freely interchanged the concepts of pleasure and enjoyment, as though they were one and the same. In fact, I did that earlier in this book; I wrote a whole chapter about pleasure and never hinted that there might be more to it. But there is.

The difference between the fleeting experience of pleasure and the focused experience of enjoyment is the difference between being a passive observer of your own life and its artist. The confusion between the two comes in part from our culture, which is fascinated with immediate gratification and markets the fleeting experience of pleasure as real happiness. Our pleasure response is brief because it comes and goes with the rise and fall of the satisfaction of our needs. Even the best of meals only satisfies deeply until hunger strikes again—that thing you *had* to have rarely offers more than momentary contentment.

Don't get me wrong, I am a big proponent of expanding our capacity for pleasure and have allowed my own hedonism many a long weekend. We used pleasure in chapter 2 as a guide into our deeper erotic soul, and it is an excellent guide—the best we have. But what is pleasure leading us *to?* To be meaningful, the journey of increasing pleasure should lead us to a true and lasting enjoyment of life. Even the holy grail of orgasmic release is a fleeting pleasure compared to the long-term joy of sharing a life with someone we love. In a heartbeat I would give up endless pleasure—orgasms, massages, the very best meals I have eaten—for the deep satisfaction and lasting happiness of discovering what makes me a better version of myself.

What is the essential difference between fleeting pleasure and lasting happiness? *Attention.* Simply put, when we focus our attention on getting better at something, on growing our abilities and interests in whatever makes us curious and feel more alive, we tap the source of lasting happiness. By combining active attention with an intention to commit ourselves fully to the things that inspire us, we immerse ourselves in the moment and the life that is in front of us. Whether your joy comes through your attention to your partner or to a beloved pursuit, like music, sports, or learning, it is the process of honing our attention that heals and grows us.

Recent social science research bears out this intimate connection between attention and lasting happiness. In a study detailed in the book *Flow*, by Mihaly Csikszentmihalyi, people reported that their most enjoyable moments occurred when they were fully immersed in activities they love to do—the sort of immersion that does not notice the passage of time or consider when the next meal will be. These moments of "flow," as they are referred to by the scientists who study them, are the gifts we get when our intention to become more of ourselves is matched by the experiences we need to grow.[1]

These moments of total absorption in what we love feel like we're being carried in the flow of life. People will often describe these experiences by saying that time "stood still," that they were one with the rock being climbed or the music they were playing. Or, as my son says about his very best games, "the basketball and the hoop were all that existed." In this magical space and time, we are fully present, and the universe enjoys us. When we are not chasing or being chased by our thousands of thoughts, which plague us with worry or attack us with self-defeating feelings of worthlessness, we find deep wholeness.

Committing to discovering and attending to your personal joy is a lifelong process of self-development. It is not easy to give yourself over to this kind of deep attention. There are many days when even the activities that we usually enjoy the most don't do anything for us, as my son will attest when he can't find his shot or the competition is too stiff. Sometimes we just can't find that place of magical attention, and the most joy we can get from an experience comes from reflecting on our goals after the bruises have healed. But working with our attention to find lasting joy is fundamentally how we show up most meaningfully in our lives—and especially in our relationships.

When I got married at nineteen, I didn't have a clue how important attention is to maintaining healthy relationships. Growing up in a dysfunctional home, all I knew about attention was that the adults around me were wrapped up in their own stories and had no time or patience for me. My longing for attention grew up with me. What I most remember of my teen years was listening endlessly to Barry Manilow, alone in my room, longing for that promise of being seen and held in the loving gaze of another. I was sure that once someone fell in love with me, I would become full and whole. Most love songs are about that longing. We long to fall in love in order to fill that empty place and to be seen.

Falling in love intoxicates with the promise of filling our need for attention. More than anything else, attention is what fills us up, makes us fully ourselves. In the early days of a romance, two people are so deeply interested in each other that every gaze feels like a warm embrace. Indeed, there may be no more healing a balm than the soft and steady reflection of loving eyes resting on our face or the sweet peace of feeling deeply heard by someone who loves us. I have come to believe that this is really all we ever want—the full presence and attention of love.

But we easily confuse the intoxicating experience of falling in love, which holds the promise of meeting our often unrecognized need for attention, with the hard work of loving someone over time. The truth is that the initial intoxication of falling in love fades; our long-term relationships are simply not capable of attending to us like this on a daily basis. I used to get so angry with my husband because I had this idea that when you married somebody, you would have that magical thing, finally—that attention that fills you, heals all your wounds, sees and accepts you completely, forever. How many of us have believed that we'll finally be forever happy once we've said "I do"? But after the honeymoon period wears off (it usually lasts six months at best), what you're left with is two people who are each dying for the attention of the other and at the same time unable to fully give their own attention.

After the honeymoon period had worn off for us, when my husband was in his last year of medical school and we had our first toddler, I came across a book at the library titled *Married to Medicine: An Intimate Portrait of Doctors' Wives*. It was a compendium of all that could, and often did, go wrong being married to a physician. The stories of affairs with nurses struck my deepest fears, and I resolved never to be the wife who turns away from her husband's sexual needs. On the whole, this was an easy commitment for me to keep as orgasm has always been enticing to me, but I also remember plenty of times in those early days when I was too tired or just wasn't interested in sex and felt obliged anyway—not by him, but by my own fear of not being there for him.

This obligatory sex was the most disappointing and lifeless sex we ever had. There is something about obligation that shuts down any possibility for our own pleasure. Feeling obligated to do anything, even activities that we might otherwise enjoy, completely drains us of desire. Obligation somehow turns activities we once found pleasant into something so uncomfortable; it can seem impossible to give them our full attention. All we can think is, "When will this be over?" We tune out of the present moment, which feels too painful, and take our attention to some silly list or a fantasy of the future. Whereas giving sex our undivided attention opens the door to pleasure, the sex we are barely present for because we feel obligated is deadening.

What's more, because curiosity and courage depend on our attention, when we come to sex out of obligation and are inattentive to what unfolds, we also lose our freedom, the freedom to choose, to explore, to engage. Early in my marriage, when I felt a heavy sense of obligation around sex, it was impossible for me to stay in the moment, and so I relied on our regular routine, my mind wandering to some unfinished to-do list or, worse still, degenerating into unspoken resentments as I waited for the sex to end. This was way before I learned how I could use fantasy as a fuel for my erotic life. And I was still missing the most critical element that determined why sex worked or fell flat for us—attention.

It took me years to begin to see that the heavy sense of obligation I felt around sex completely vanished when I had the courage to be curious about my experience and to fully attend to it, no matter what. The early years of our marriage were shaped by my deep needs to be seen and valued, needs that were competing with the needs that my husband brought from his own childhood. During our many years of couples therapy, the issue of attention dominated our inability to communicate and connect, especially as our family grew and demanded even more of our attention. I still remember the therapy session when I first really understood what attention meant to each of us and that inattention was not a personal attack but rather the reality of our busy lives. The reality of our growing family was that there were often more demands than resources when it came to our collective attention, but no one was to blame for this reality. This recognition brought a softening to our old unresolved anger, and it also was my first clue to the freedom and capacity I could develop with my own attention.

The struggle I experienced in my own relationship is just one example of the way many relationships falter early on because attention is not fully understood. It seems like giving our full attention to the people we love should be natural and effortless. But consider the times you've spent with a child, how difficult it is to be fully present, without any distractions. For me, in all the years of raising children, sustaining this kind of presence was a constant quest—and that I didn't give my kids enough of my attention is the thing I most regret. Driving my kids to and from the music lessons, soccer games, dance practices, I believed that my choice to be self-employed was a privilege and a gift for them. And yet as years passed, they told me more than once, "Yeah, you were there, but you were always on your phone." Ouch! I know that my inability to attend, to choose to truly attend to the person or moment in front of me, speaks louder than words about the priority I give them.

We are not truly *giving* our attention when we are doing three things simultaneously. We are not giving our attention when we are struggling with our own pain, fear, and insecurities. We are not able to offer attention to anyone when we are judging them. Half our attention is not experienced as half; it is experienced as complete absence. Simone Weil wrote, "Attention is the rarest and purest form of generosity."[2] Just as true generosity is an act of giving that has no strings attached, true attention is an act of offering your fullest presence to the person and moment you are with, exactly as they are.

Why is it so hard to offer someone, even someone we love dearly, our undivided attention? I've asked myself this question countless times, and the answer, I'm now convinced, is that our attention for others comes from a pool of our own that we are given when we are children. When we give our attention, we give from the pool of love we've received. To the extent that we were attended to as children, we will more effortlessly be able to attend to ourselves and to others. To the extent that we were not attended to, we tend to hoard our attention. We are like people who lived through the Depression; later, when they have enough money, or even an abundance of money, they may still feel like there's never enough, as if at any moment they could go back to that place of lack. The same is true of attention. If we have grown up without enough, then later, even when we are surrounded by those we love and who love us, we may be haunted by the feeling that we are not being seen or that at any moment we'll be forgotten about or pushed to the side. As a mother, when I would work to recognize my kids so that they felt seen and witnessed, it would often provoke the old feelings of absence and invisibility that grew up in me.

Thankfully, it is possible to practice and develop our capacity for attention. Even if we were not attended to as children—and many of us were not—we can learn how to open up our attention and bring our full awareness into our relationships. This is an essential practice. Truly, your attention is the most powerful agent of change that you can bring to your relationship. Consider how you attend to the details of your financial life or your career; your intimate relationships deserve at least that much of your daily attention. Not surprisingly, over time, the number one thing that harms relationships? Inattentiveness. It may manifest as inattentiveness to our partner, but more deeply, it is inattentiveness to our own wounds, which generates a broader inattentiveness that leaves us incapable of discerning what our true responsibility is to our relationships.

This bears repeating: our ability to pay attention to those we love always begins with our ability to attend to ourselves. If we never enjoyed the undivided, loving attention of the important adults in our life, we also likely never learned how to pay attention to ourselves—how to listen for or recognize our own thoughts, feelings, and achievements. When we feel starved for attention from others, what we are actually missing is our own attention, our own presence.

>> A great practice for developing our capacity for attending to ourselves is simple, but not easy. It involves learning to pay attention to yourself by listening to your own thoughts. All you need is any type of wristband or bracelet that's easy to put on and take off. Each time you witness yourself having disparaging thoughts about yourself, switch the wristband to the other wrist. The effort to switch your wristband is enough to slow your thinking down so that your mind can come up with something more constructive.

Don't be surprised or discouraged by how many negative thoughts pervade your thinking at first. The more you pay attention, the more your mind will replace those useless thoughts with more neutral observations and eventually with supportive, positive thinking.

One of the biggest gifts that the loving attention of others gives us is the awareness and experience of our own presence. Love transmitted and received through attention transforms the inner landscape, replacing our emotional needs with a sense of self-esteem and sufficiency.

This learning is critical because when we feel like we both *have* and *are* enough, we gain the space and capacity to pay attention to others. It has taken me decades to become aware of how my childhood attention deficit compromised my ability to both give and receive my own attention.

Raising my four kids provided endless opportunities for me to notice when I had given away more attention than I had stored in my own pool. And I know I am not alone with this very common female scenario, as women are both innately inclined and subconsciously trained to give away our attention to everyone and everything else around us. It wasn't until the event that's now known in my family as the Infamous Plate-Throwing Dinner that the deep imbalance in my ability to listen for my own needs became obvious to me—and everyone in my family.

Until I started throwing dinner plates that night, I had no idea how depleted I had become. I was so busy mindlessly attending to the needs of others—kids, coworkers, my husband, friends and acquaintances—that it never occurred to me to listen for the neglect and pain I was experiencing so acutely inside. And then, suddenly, I saw myself, not serving dinner to my family, but flinging plates of it through the air.

Now I realize that my inability to listen for my own suffering was partly due to how very difficult, and often frightening, it can be to listen to ourselves. All the little annoyances and pent-up frustrations that I had been ignoring for so long came crashing down that night at dinner. Not listening and later acting out our overwhelming need for attention is dangerous—not only because plates will fly but also because all the feelings that we suppress and refuse to acknowledge take on a life of their own inside us, devolving into a cacophony of anxiety and insecurity and preventing us from believing in or even recognizing our best self.

The longer we go not paying attention to ourselves, the more entrapped we become in the stories that arise from these unattended parts of ourselves. The tragedy of this lowly place is that we not only lose the ability to pay attention to our own needs but also become completely unavailable to those we love.

When I'm in a cycle of breakdown, my internal four-year-old loses control and, overcome with feelings of depletion and neglect, acts out, as I did that night with the dinner plates. That night was a life turning point for me. Afterward, I became committed to both listening inside and creating spaces to vent and release what I had spent so long keeping bottled up. I began by creating a plate-throwing gallery in my backyard. Putting together a cinder block wall and collecting a stack of cheap secondhand plates became a therapeutic story revision of my dinnertime breakdown. It created levity and normalized what I needed to express. (My kids thought it was nuts—until they threw a couple of plates themselves.) Giving myself permission to pay attention to and express my pent-up feelings allowed me to listen to the many younger versions of myself, each of whom had been screaming for my attention over the years. As I learned to listen more deeply and pay more attention inside, the light of my attention decreased my self-judgment and increased my self-trust. For the first time in my life, I began to experience myself as loveable.

>> When you feel frustrated, give yourself permission to feel your pent-up feelings. You don't have to build a wall to throw plates against, but notice if, in being attended to, your frustration wants to express itself in some outer, physical way. Feel the energy of your internal four-year-old; is there a way you can release this energy through play? (After all, we're talking about a four-year-old.) Release your frustrated energy through physical movement: do a hard workout at the gym, dance, or take a brisk walk, even adding some sprints. Or better still, take your inner child to the park and play; tire yourself out the way kids do. The key is to allow yourself to feel everything and not to judge yourself for how you are feeling.

Our sense of being lovable (or not) is a deep part of the personal narrative that comes to us in bits and pieces over the course of many years growing up. But this personal narrative is more malleable than most people realize, and we can transform it by engaging with the stories we tell. Our personal narrative is like a road map, and shifting its course internally is like changing worlds. So listen without judgment to the stories that you are telling yourself and then suggest new ones. Let yourself become more loving toward yourself. All of those stories and all of those anxieties are, after all, just thoughts, your mind's attempt to look out for you. Yet sometimes we have to teach ourselves what's best for us.

It's so important to give our attention to our inner lives in this way because when we don't listen to our own stories or understand our own needs, we are stuck inside ourselves, unable to see our needs and therefore trapped by them. We expect our partner to take care of us, but we don't even know what we need ourselves. We may tell ourselves that we are being selfish, that we should always be thinking about our partner, but often this is just a way of circling back to our own unexplored needs to feel loved and appreciated: Does he like what *I've* cooked? Is she happy with *me?* Bringing our attention as a gentle witness to the old story lines of our insecurities and judgment is the courageous path of releasing them. Your own needs are the knot that you need to unravel before you can bring your full attention to anyone else.

Even as I gained more skills in listening for and attending to my own needs, there were still many times over the years when I felt unable to meet my needs or those of my partner and my kids. I would get stuck in old patterns, not sure whose needs should prevail. Over and over it was like losing my way; I felt both unable to recognize my own needs and to discern what my true responsibility was to my relationship. I would still sometimes come up against a powerful longing for an unbiased, unconditional witness—attention I felt I wasn't getting in my relationship. I didn't know where to go with this longing until I interviewed Dr. Stan Tatkin, author of *Wired for Love*. It was only then that this seemingly unsolvable relationship puzzle started to fit together.

The missing piece when it comes to both sustaining and growing an intimate relationship is that the focus of your attention cannot be on your own needs or even your partner's needs. It must be on the needs of *the relationship itself*. For many it is a radical leap to recognize that when you focus your attention, not on your own needs or your partner's needs but on the needs of the relationship, you produce the paradoxical effect of getting your needs met in a way that they could never be met by making them primary. It's not about what I need or what you need, but what the *container* needs to hold both of us. This is where attention becomes a magical dance of reciprocity: when both partners pour their loving attention into the container of their relationship, together they build a foundation of strength and a pure space of acceptance that could never have come from their separate attempts to meet their own needs. (See "Further Reading and Resources" for more about Tatkin's book.)

In my own marriage, I have found that focusing on the needs of the container works. When I insist on my own needs, it usually only makes things worse, not only because I am not getting what I want but also because my insistence on me doesn't support the container of the relationship I hold dear. When I can say instead, "I don't know how to make this relationship big enough to hold what we both want," a very different conversation can happen. By reflecting on what's missing for me in terms of the bigger relationship, I'm not asking anybody to be different to please me but focusing instead on the container that we're building for all of us. I know that it is only by strengthening the container that holds us that we can all get our needs met.

And yet this knowing demands both practice and time. It begins with asking questions like, "How can I feed this thing that we both need? How can I give this thing the support it needs to grow? What does the relationship need so that it can survive all the challenges that are sure to come?" As you begin to shift your attention to the health of the relationship container, it gets easier to trust the relationship as a real, living thing. You trust that the bond is bigger than the challenges, trust in the life and history of the relationship.

What's more, conceiving of the relationship as a living entity that's separate from the people it contains also lets you observe how that entity is changing over time. The wonderful effect of this is that it makes everything less personal; the work becomes about healing the relationship, not healing or changing the individuals. It gives you both a break when you can realize there's a third thing that's living between you. Think of the container as being made of both partners' strengths, weaknesses, and insecurities; wanting to heal the container gets you both off the hook personally and therefore allows you both to heal, in ways that you never could by yourself.

Focusing your attention on the container also has the effect of bringing you together, making you deeply part of each other's lives. Through the container of the relationship, you participate in each other's personal changes, whereas without it, you are separate individuals, cut off from each other and without a common, living bond. The relationship becomes a place where you both consent to care for this thing that's bigger than the two of you separately.

Most people don't grow up knowing that it's the relationship, not the individuals, that needs to be attended to. And even when we get to adulthood, it's not obvious. We keep thinking, "I have to change" or "He has to change," when in fact, for the relationship to work, and therefore for sex to work, it's the relationship that has to change. When you stop worrying about my needs or your needs and instead give your attention to the relationship, the whole dynamic changes. It becomes a conversation about sustaining an atmosphere hospitable to love.

Just as there are clear, concrete things we can do to sustain the natural environment—recycling, driving less and walking more, supporting organic agriculture—there are things we can do to create and sustain an atmosphere of love for the container of our relationship. I find it helpful to describe these things by drawing on language we use to talk about the ecological system that sustains life. Cultivating this atmosphere is like caring for a garden. We can't *make* a garden grow, but when we provide pure water, rich soil, and fresh air, we create the right conditions for it to grow. In the same way, the atmosphere in which love thrives can be clarified and cared for. Just as small daily acts of caring can add up over time to a beautiful, flourishing garden, daily loving acts can create a space in which a relationship can truly thrive.

So how do we create a healthy, loving atmosphere for our relationships? The rich soil, pure water, and fresh air that our relationships need are attention to our *thinking*, attention to how we spend our *time*, and attention to *how we communicate* with each other. Let's take a look at how nurturing each aspect can deepen our ability to be sexual.

ENRICHING THE SOIL: SAYING YES

Sustaining an atmosphere hospitable to love starts with *how we think*, both when we are with our partner and when we are alone. Our thoughts are incredibly powerful: they keep us connected or they drive us apart. But when was the last time you noticed the emotional quality of your thoughts about yourself? Your partner? What about the emotional quality of your thoughts about your relationship, the atmosphere you create together? The soil that will allow your relationship to thrive is your own thinking, and the quality of that soil depends on how much attention you give it.

It is strange to consider how frequently we don't recognize both the quality of our thoughts or the power of our thinking when it comes to our intimate relationships. How we think is incredibly powerful: the thoughts we choose and cultivate literally keep us connected to our partner or drive us apart. And it isn't just in terms of our relationships that we don't pay attention to our thinking; we also tune out to our habitual thoughts about ourselves. Most people follow the 80-20 rule when it comes to their thinking—80 percent of their thoughts are consistently negative about some aspect of their lives. It is impossible to thrive or to grow in a life dominated by a negative-feedback loop. And it is no wonder that so many of us struggle to feel the love coming toward us when we are forever on a negative train of thought that prevents us from witnessing and believing in the love that's right in front of us.

One profound impact that negative thinking has in our relationships is the way that it makes doubt the leader. Especially when it comes to intimacy, we question what we are doing, and in this space of doubt—often without realizing—we put one foot out the door. So many relationships suffer a premature demise because one (or both) of the partners is inventing an exit strategy rather than fully committing to the person and relationship they are in. The tragedy of having one foot out the door is that a relationship can never really evolve unless both people have both feet in. You don't ever really get to see what your relationship can become if you or your partner keeps one foot out the door. When both partners are engaged and really committed to sustaining the living entity that connects them, it is an entirely different relationship—one that you can't even imagine when you are busy holding the door ajar with one foot.

Changing your thinking starts with a simple willingness to pay attention to your thoughts. We can't just push our negative thoughts away, but often, just bringing our active attention to them acts to short-circuit our habitual negative thinking, giving us space in which we can replace the negative with thoughts that are more positive (or at least neutral) about the relationship. We go from habitually saying no to creating the space in which we can begin to say yes.

The work of saying yes and bringing our self fully into our relationship goes way beyond merely coexisting or cohabiting. It is easy for couples to confuse coexisting with truly showing up for each other. Coexisting and truly showing up appear the same when we grow accustomed to not allowing ourselves to need and be needed. Yet coexisting doesn't have any of the staying power that truly showing up does because it happens out of habit, not choice. Couples who coexist eat cereal at the same table and brush their teeth in the same sink, but coordinated hygiene isn't a bond.

Saying yes doesn't mean constant dates (although every now and again it is nice to take time away). Rather, it means, creating an atmosphere of togetherness through small acts on a daily basis. Instead of reading the paper, offer to help with dinner. Sharing a funny story, recounting part of your day, or offering to listen to your partner's day is a more sustainable choice than putting on the television.

Often, saying yes means simply attending to our own thoughts and not acting on the basis of the negative ones. At the very least, we can learn to insert a pause between a negative thought and a habitual reaction. Just by giving yourself time to take a few breaths before responding slows down the mind and gives it a chance to choose a different route. Giving yourself more time between the issues that trigger you and your response is often all you need to start a new line of thinking.

When you are doing the work of cultivating positive thoughts about your relationship, these small acts emerge naturally from that soil, like the first shoots of your garden.

PURE WATER: SPENDING TIME

Our attention is always a reflection of what we do with our time. Being truly attentive might mean spending more time when you would ordinarily rush or gloss over the details. It can also mean *creating* time to spend with another. There's a quote, usually attributed to Lao Tzu, that I love: "Time is a created thing. To say 'I don't have time' is like saying 'I don't want to.'" Truly showing up in your relationship, moment by moment, even during the mundane activities, creates safety in every other part of your relationship, including the erotic parts. When we feel safe, we explore more. As we are able to become more curious, we also become more open to experiencing pleasure. Relationship growth is a capital investment in time, but without that investment, connections can't deepen. It is easy, in this era of instant connectivity, to lose sight of what it means to commit to the real face time love demands.

How much time you make for love is a deeply meaningful measure of the health and sustainability of your relationship. This is especially true when you consider the outrageous scheduling demands that we agree to without hesitation for our work lives, our children's activity calendar, or our favorite social media connections. In the midst of these demands, we struggle to make time for what we know is important. Why? What makes scheduling the best hours of our intimate life so difficult? Inattentiveness—to how we are feeling, to how we are living, to how we are loving.

In part, "scheduling" and "intimacy" still seem mutually exclusive even for couples in committed relationships. Many of us still believe that good sex can only happen when it occurs spontaneously, and somehow the idea of planning it makes it less sexy, tainted with neediness no one wants to own. Deeper still are the vestiges of shame and guilt that we must confront when we actively plan our sex life. It isn't just the thrill we miss, like when we were teenagers on the couch, sneaking whatever we could get before our parents came home. It is a lack of responsibility for our erotic selves that often keeps us from planning time for sex, which demands that we claim the most unpredictable and, to some degree, uncontrollable parts of ourselves. And yet, befriending our erotic selves and planning lovemaking amidst our regularly scheduled events bodes well for both the health and longevity of the body as well as the soul of the relationship.

For many years when our kids were small, my husband and I would save lovemaking for after the last thing on the list was done. Arriving at our bedroom at our lowest ebb of energy after the kids were in bed, the bills were paid, and all the lights turned off often made the prospect of sex feel more like a chore than the deep release that I should have known from memory was a worthy trade for sleep. Trying to fit sex into tiny slivers of our time wasn't successful in creating the spontaneous connection we felt was missing. Too often the exhausted late-night energy was not enough to get us through the learning we were still doing about how to find pleasure together.

Once we started to plan lovemaking dates, even the random late-night interludes got more exciting. One sex date we had on a sunny afternoon (we'd arranged for a babysitter) was so passionate because it was so different from our regular routine. Even the smallest changes of time and venue that your full attention can bring to a withering sex life are remarkable, because making and fulfilling a love plan shows your partner that you are all in.

FRESH AIR: CLEAR COMMUNICATION

When we listen with our entire body, we bring a great healing balm to our relationships. One of the most reliable techniques for teaching aspiring actors how to "fall in love" on screen is to use the power of this kind of full-body attention. Even in play acting, fully focusing our attention on someone feels like love, whether it is true or not. We witness attentiveness as love perhaps nowhere more deeply than in the experience of feeling truly heard.

One of my favorite quotes and one that often comes to mind when I fall deeply into conversation with my beloved friends is, "I felt it shelter to speak with you."[3] For me it is a feeling of being held in a safe, soft container, where the communication is happening in part through our words, but even when I misspeak or can't find the right words, there is an essence of my being heard. This experience is so healing that it is arguably one of the most profound examples of love acting as a verb. And it is also in this deep, attentive listening that the currency of air flows through your relationship, providing the perfect atmosphere to kindle physical intimacy.

For many couples, this art of listening has yet to be fully realized. For one thing, different people have different styles of communicating. For example, where my husband is a man of few words, I know my feelings and thoughts most clearly when I express them. Understanding these differences between us, and knowing that they are not personal, helps us to engage more amicably. Recognizing and naming the key differences in your communication styles creates an agreed upon buffer zone so that you don't take each other so personally.

Bringing in fresh air to sustain the container sometimes means engaging in conversations that may not be particularly interesting to you but that promote an atmosphere hospitable to love. The willingness to listen—to things that don't interest you or that you might not be able to fix or change—sends the message to your partner that you care, that you have their back no matter what. What's more, listening in this way—without trying to solve the other person's problems or to steer the conversation—provides the space for the other person to figure out their own solutions. This space is a true shelter for love, and having it grows the confidence not only of the partner being heard but also of the container itself.

Over time, as my husband and I learned the power of this kind of attentive listening, we used our new understanding to enliven our intimate connection. At first it was the coining of code words that we would insert in the lists of pick-ups and drop-offs for the day. It was like learning how to flirt again, and it got me reserving my energy for our time together. Setting these dates to be together became a kind of foreplay that kept a sexual current alive between us. I needed the vital glue that the promise of his intimate attention offered me. Part permission to fantasize and part a genuine interest in my sex appeal, his interest and mine let us connect even in the most trying of times.

The more we explored and got creative with our invented language for our intimate lives, the easier it was to carve out times in the week to spend together intimately, and the better the sex got. The challenging issues of initiating—who asked whom, who said yes or no—faded as the intrigue of our game and the quality of our two-feet-in sex grew. We were more playful together, and when tempers flared over stupid household details, we knew we were overdue for another sex date. Setting up times for regular lovemaking and cultivating a language of pleasure with your partner is the most powerful message of love you can send.

As vital as listening is, both *what* we express and the *tone* with which we express it weigh in just as heavily. Many people speak to their partners on a regular basis in a way that they wouldn't speak with a stranger. Often the tone of voice we use says more about our intention than the words themselves. Sarcasm or telling jokes at our partner's expense is not funny. It erodes all of the hard work you have both done to make the container you share safe, and it eliminates the possibility of building an erotic language together. How you communicate your feelings and desires, not just erotically but in every way, is how you connect with your partner. When we give our full attention to what and how we are speaking to someone else, and to fully receiving their response, we are creating a live current of energetic possibility.

Combining this with the freedom to take responsibility for our *own* erotic needs and desires makes for life-changing conversations. When we are willing to talk about our sexual life, we open a whole expanse of possibility that never existed before. For many people, speaking honestly and openly about desire, or the lack of it, is the passage out of what may have been taboo for way too long. What's more, developing a language for love is one of the strongest predictors of having a good sex life. Couples who can talk about what they want or prefer in their physical intimacy are often able to get it, or at least move closer to it.

The transcendent, unifying effect of focusing on the container of the relationship is especially important when it comes to sex. In my work as a loveologist, I've come to believe that the primary reason so many sexual relationships are a mess is that people can't ask for what they need sexually (or don't even know what they need). They have a load of needs they can't identify or name, and they expect their partner to somehow do this work for them! I say this with full recognition that when I began my marriage at the young age of nineteen, I was just as inarticulate and confused.

Therefore, it is so important to begin this work by attending to ourselves, recognizing our thought patterns and hearing them out, but not getting pulled into the story so that we continue to act out the same dysfunctional patterns. The key is to widen our attention from our own individual needs to those of the relationship, which contains both partners in a loving atmosphere and which will ultimately nourish both partners' needs. This widening of attention requires a deliberate leap. It takes a lot of maturity to make that leap, but that leap is vital for sustaining a relationship. It will work if you trust that by taking care of what holds you, you will be taking care of yourself. Trust that you're creating something that's unique, that lives and breathes in the world because both people continue to say yes to it.

When we have that trust, there is a new power in bringing our loving attention—which is nonjudgmental, soft, and accepting—to our partner. Giving our partner our loving, full attention can be a sexual act. Coming into bed with a head full of thoughts, any kind of thoughts, from to-do lists to insecurities to anticipation, will prevent you from the experience of engaging sex. Good sex demands one thing above all: your full presence. And orgasm specifically is impossible to achieve when your brain is busy processing some list or anxiously reviewing your day.

So how do we fully arrive in the arms of a lover, empty of our mental noise and capable of the giving and receiving that make sex so compelling? It helps to create a practice of emptying our mind, a daily moment of bearing witness not only to the nonstop flow of errant thoughts that disrupt our attention but also, and more importantly, to the hot, sticky emotional ties that bind us invisibly. We don't often link this meditative work to passionate sex, yet there may be no more powerful part of our sexual anatomy to engage than a brain that can settle down into calm awareness. Showing up to our love lives, emptied of our cares and concerns, means becoming an empty vessel that love can fill.

>> Start slowly in filling the empty space between you and your partner. Explore aspects of intimacy by breaking them down into the smallest elements. For example, when thinking of the kiss, reflect on how lips, tongue, and the space between you make the dance of physical communication erotic. Respecting the space between you as a crucial aspect of any approach not only slows down the process but also affirms the delicate connections that give sex its buzz.

Even if you aren't emotionally engaged for the long haul in the sexual relationship you are playing in, have the courage to allow yourself to feel what is being exchanged in the depth of intimacy. So much harm comes after casual sex when people cut themselves off from the feelings in their body. Our feelings reflect the barometer of our sense of safety, of being seen and valued. Sex that we do not allow to engage our hearts shuts them down.

Healing our erotic lives begins with fully engaging our attention and our hearts in an interactive and informative dialogue. The mysterious and often shattered connection between our capacity for desire and sexual arousal is repaired in these empathetic exchanges. Our erotic soul awakens when we focus and connect our visceral attention to the entire range of our sensory experience. Sexual intimacy is the singular human act that heals and brings together the emotional, physical, mental, and spiritual bodies into a unified whole. When we are whole and connected, we are capable of experiencing a form of gratitude that is not just a thought, but also a visceral response. Like joy and pleasure, gratitude acts as a creative burst of energy that springs from us, with a single purpose, to do good—to be more fully ourselves, fully present. As we learn to embody gratitude, our heart cracks wide open and fills us up. We are loved. We are able to love.

9

GRATITUDE

Good sex with someone you love, and who loves you, is a pure, ecstatic experience of gratitude. This kind of gratitude isn't the cerebral "counting your blessings" kind of gratitude. It is felt throughout the body. It is a feeling of fullness that is a thank you. Grateful sex is the visceral experience of true sexual freedom.

There are times after I make love to my husband that I wished I had made a video so that I would always be able to remember how crazy and intense and out of our minds we were in the throes of passion. Even a few hours later, my memories of sex take on the quality of dreams, and describing the sensation or even the sequence starts to feel like sand running through my fingers. When I mention the idea of filming us to him, he scoffs at the idea—partly because he would be mortified to have such a private and essential part of our relationship recorded, and partly because it would be so weird to do it. But then I imagine in twenty years, or maybe less, one of us gone and how happy the other would be to see us again. I can just see myself, masturbating and sobbing all the while, wishing for just one more time and kicking myself that I didn't appreciate the wonder of our lovemaking more when I had it. The truth is that most times, after we are intimate, I only have to hold the thought "What if that was the last time?" for a moment before tears well up in my eyes.

The revelation of our erotic selves is an overwhelming awakening, even and especially after decades of knowing someone. The act of fully abandoning my consciousness into the mysterious sexual spaces that dwell outside of language, the nuances of what we do with and to each other, blows my mind every time. The power of the sensation and pleasure evoked by human sexual ecstasy is singular in all the world. Every year I get multiple emails about events that are planned to inspire as many lovers as possible worldwide to orgasm at the same moment with the intention of sending that collective ecstatic energy toward universal healing. I don't know if I have ever hit the prescribed time slot, but the idea of healing comes to me often when I am making love. It makes me wonder if the potent emotional pain I expel during sex is from lifetimes ago, or if I am just beginning to tap into the lives of the millions of women who are living right now in terror and pain because of the trauma and fear that haunt so much of human sexuality. In many places in the world, being born female is practically criminal. How are the daughters of so many fathers, the sisters of so many brothers, not cherished or protected?

The torment of sexual trauma and pain has eclipsed our planet so many times that it now exists like a layer that touches us all. It is safe to say that at any given moment, there are tragically at least as many, if not more, sexual acts that are committed in violence and aggression as those created out of love. The resulting sexual terror and shame pervade the essence of human sexuality in sometimes invisible ways, cutting us off from our own desire, each other, and the divine. And it makes those of us who are blessed enough to create and participate in loving sexual acts responsible for sharing that love with those who are less fortunate. This sharing is the first step in healing the pain and terror of sex so that our inherent human sexuality is no longer a source of suffering but of pleasure and lasting joy.

It starts with being deeply grateful for each and every moment of erotic bliss we get. No taking our love for granted. No dismissing the wonder of physical intimacy and the emotional cleansing that only deep lovemaking generates. This is one of the most powerful forms of gratitude, sourced from the energy of our rapture, which we can embody and offer to others. Like a prayer, our loving sexual relationships are a potent remedy for the immense body of pain dominating our collective sexual consciousness.

It wasn't always like this for me. For much of my life I didn't experience this kind of gratitude—in sex or anywhere else in my life. My expressions of thankfulness often felt hollow, qualified with feeling beholden, questioning my own worth. It wasn't until I began to wonder why I couldn't evoke the kind of visceral gratitude I would often read about as a source of positivity that it became clear to me: I had never been able to feel this kind of gratitude because I had never learned how to *receive*.

In this, I am far from alone. In my own family, the capacity to receive was never even an idea. My father, right up to the end of his life, could not accept help, let alone love, of any kind. Partly due to fear of being dependent on anyone, partly to feeling unworthy of love, his inability to receive kept him out of love's reach, no matter how I much I tried to give to him, until the day he died alone. Witnessing the consequences of his choices convinced me just how important it is to follow an active path to receiving the good in life. Simultaneously letting go of past experiences, especially the painful ones, and opening up to receive the full range of our present experience is really the only way to access gratitude.

As I focused on becoming a receiver, I was stunned by how much goodness started coming to me so easily. Having spent so many years trying to make things happen, I found it scary to let go and really trust that good things could come my way, unbidden. For much of my life I felt compelled to push the river, my focus stuck on where it wasn't working. In ways that weren't always obvious to me, my driven goal setting was an obsession with trying to make things turn out the way I wanted. Consumed by the ways I thought things should happen, and trying to control other people's perceptions about what was happening, I spent years without room to receive much of anything.

Paradoxically (why is it that spiritual growth seems always to begin with a paradox?), to be receptive to love, we first have to learn how to let go. Unfortunately, the time and culture in which we are living do not make letting go easy. As we live in a culture that values material possessions and their accumulation, it is easy to believe that what we own defines our life. Often the richest lives are created by people who strive not to accumulate more but to *be* more. Our ability to accept what is and to let go of how we think things should be leaves room for what matters most, and it fosters our ability to become more of ourselves. Letting go, the sister of receiving, teaches that sometimes there is a more powerful force than trying. Effort and aspiration are balanced by having the courage and insight to let go.

This practice of letting go in the service of connecting with ourselves and with others heals in concentric circles, starting with our own life and radiating out. It is an immensely rewarding path, but not an easy one. As I have shared throughout this book, learning to feel has been a challenging journey that has required opening up to the full range of my experience, including the most uncomfortable aspects. There have been days when going to these painful places has felt like more than I could do. Yet, as time passes and I keep opening, this practice of receiving through letting go has transformed not only my outer exchanges with the world but even more deeply the way I live in my body.

All the ways we break down, whether physical, emotional, or mental, are contained in this amazing temple called our body. The broken places are the treasure troves of our life's work and deserve our gratitude, too. Usually we reserve feelings of gratitude for the things we love, but when we have the courage to offer a small slice of our grateful attention to the most painful places, we welcome them back into ourselves and become more whole. Gratitude for our broken places always translates into more courage, more patience, and more humor, too. Gratitude is at its most powerful when it lightens our load by transmuting our pain into compassion.

Gratitude is also often the missing element for healing old emotional wounds that our bodies hold onto. The body is at once the container for unresolved emotions and the vehicle for transmuting them into wisdom. Bodies do not lie; they record precisely and then store the information, waiting for us to pay attention. If we don't pay attention, what is recorded hardens in us and turns into disease of one kind or another. This hardening easily becomes a difficult habit to break because it impacts the heart, mind, and body in equal proportion. We don't see that it is through this habit of hardening that we become rigid, our emotional tension solidifies into a limited range of motion, and we cement our feelings and even fleeting perceptions into intractable judgments. We lose touch with the fluid and spacious beings we truly are. Memories of childhood, when movement was effortless and happiness was sensory, feel like something imagined rather than a real connection to who we were.

This hardening offers the most accurate picture of the aging process, too. It is easy to stop moving the painful places in the body, believing that this motionless space will heal if we leave it alone. Yet the less we move the painful places, the stiffer and more intractable the pain becomes. Gently coaxing ourselves to maintain exercise routines when we are in pain is one way we learn to live peaceably with weakness and teach our heart how strong we are, especially when we are wounded.

An old French proverb says, "Gratitude is the memory of the heart." It is a golden and rare moment when our hearts can teach us how to feel our pain and grief, how to befriend our fears, by experiencing what we have with the life-changing force of gratitude. With gratitude we are able to move beyond our once-rigid boundaries to deeply connect with others and, most importantly, with ourselves. Letting go of the old emotional wounds that our bodies hold on to is gratitude embodied. By releasing our grip on old pain, we free our hands to receive the love and pleasure coming toward us. This is really where grateful sex—sex that works—begins.

So, you may be thinking, if this is where sex that works begins, then why is "Gratitude" the last chapter of this book, not the first?

I've made "Gratitude" the last chapter because I have found that a sense of deep gratitude is the natural culmination of each step in the process of learning to feel. It begins with the true *freedom* of taking responsibility for our thoughts and actions and committing to loving ourselves, with gratitude for all of our strengths and weaknesses. We can then bring this independence to our relationships: when nobody is being blamed and nobody is being held responsible for somebody else's pleasure, and both partners feel safe and mutually respected within the container of their relationship, then both partners have the freedom to be as they are. Grateful sex is the visceral experience of true sexual freedom, and it is the sex that brings the most *pleasure*, both physical and spiritual. In moments of grateful pleasure, giving and receiving are truly one and the same.

An experience like this of deep physical and spiritual pleasure makes accepting ourselves possible; we begin to acknowledge and let go of our old fears about what is sexually *normal* or not and to live the truth of our own experience, however that may look. Having the *courage* to gratefully embrace our unique human capacities to sense the world brings life into clear focus, decreasing the distractions that distance us from deeply feeling life's sweetest moments. With *curiosity*, and aided by courage, we open up to more and more of these moments, receiving experience without holding on or pushing away. Open and receptive, we can fully inhabit our bodies and their myriad *sensations*, which gives us access to more joy and pleasure in everyday experiences.

Bringing our full *attention* to any of our experiences, whether they are unfolding as fantasies in our minds or in three-dimensional reality, and no matter how intense they might be, is deeply healing. I know I have said this already, but it bears repeating a thousand times: nothing is more healing than your own attention. Attention makes us whole; when we are whole, we can fully embody our experience, receiving what comes and letting ourselves directly experience all of life.

>> To see just how intimately connected gratitude is with the process of learning to feel, think about the last time you felt profoundly grateful. Try to remember how it felt in your body the last time you were fully aware of how good life can be. Notice how engaged you were by your senses—whether it was the extraordinary taste of favorite foods, the scent in the early morning as one season slipped into another, the way great music changed your physiology, or the way colors captured your imagination. Spend some time savoring this remembered, grateful space.

Elicit and re-experience the fullness of your senses. Gratitude lives through our bodies. By remembering and cherishing a time in the past when you were profoundly grateful, you can summon a felt sense of gratitude anytime, any place. Gratitude makes us more intimate with our own experience, and it happens spontaneously, in the midst of any experience, when we bring our attention closer to our feelings and our senses.

Getting to sex that works, and keeping it working, depends upon our ability to remain receptive, fully present with our partner, grateful for all that transpires in this erotic space. One powerful way to visualize receiving love is to imagine yourself as a worthy physical container of love. Inevitably when you go inside to inspect this beautiful chalice, you will see that many of the erroneous beliefs you have held about yourself and others have created cracks that leak out the essence of your lovability. Taking the time to repair and patch the cracks in the container is worth the effort, as your willingness to witness and experience the pain of your own beliefs allows them to fall away. You realize that you are innately capable of receiving and holding the love that comes toward you.

When we receive love in this way, we are actually participating in a transmission of goodness. Each loving act that we receive has the power to both awaken the seed of goodness that lives in each of us and transform us into our best selves. In this receiving, gratitude becomes a visceral experience of love that wakes us up to our birthright, our own seed of loveliness, which is the truest thing about us. Gratitude embodied turns this ability to feel loved into ever-larger circles of kindness. Buddhists teach loving kindness as a fundamental practice for both inner and outer peace. In fact, all religions hold kindness as one of the central tenets of living well. "Do unto others as you would have them do unto you."

The practice of grateful kindness can happen in the smallest of gestures of support—a quiet look of understanding, a gentle tone of voice, an outstretched hand. Kindness creates space for forgiveness and letting go to occur. Acting with kindness is also a reliable balancer of mood and temper, which pulls us closer to our own center, letting us be available for the many small moments of gratitude we can overlook when we are distracted. My marriage has survived on small acts of kindness, where our friendship with each other is the leader. Not only have we been able to overcome many problems that individually we couldn't manage, but also the practice of caring about the container that holds us has made our relationship reliable and safe, which in turn has created a trustworthy pathway for us to explore a passionate, evolving sex life. Our real nakedness comes not in taking off our clothes together, but in letting down our emotional guards. Unguarded, in these moments of true presence, we cannot help but feel—and learn to feel more deeply.

Every now and again life offers you the gift of true presence. Often it is when you are faced with the stark realization of the fragility of life in a moment of loss or a miraculous reprieve. This is when your ability to embrace the moment, in this body, with this person you love, is all you need to experience the deep gratitude that changes how you *feel* the experience of your life. In these moments of pure presence, the details of life fall away, and the mystery of your frail human form and relationships is all that you have—all that you ever had.

For me, this space of full heart presence is usually stirred and accompanied by grief. Yet the more attention I can bring to the beauty and truth of my grief, the more resounding are my feelings of gratitude. When you allow yourself to befriend loss and know it for the lifelong companion that it is, you would have to be a fool to not recognize how blessed you are—for all the many ways life is working right in this moment and, even more so, for all the people that you love and have ever loved. This is, in fact, what it means to grow up or at least to grow old: to acknowledge that loss is the inevitable outcome when we love.

Loss and grief are not just consequences of death; they live in us just as deeply when relationships end, friendships wither, homes burn down. We have and we let go; that is the nature of love. And for better or worse, the more we love, the more we have to lose. Ironically, it is when we willingly dive into this vast sea of loss that we tap into the most vibrant and heartfelt experience of being alive. Our attention, our feelings of courage and gratitude, are not just thoughts then; they sing in our viscera. Perhaps the most intimate and memorable dances we share with those we love occur in this fragile, tender space in which gratitude and grief are enfolded as one in our heart.

This naked place of pure presence is not an easy one to live in. We know in these moments of pure love and connection, pure loss and loneliness, that our emotions are not thoughts in our head, but physical forces that fill our body so completely that they alter our senses. This is why falling in or out of love is a full-body experience—one that impacts how we feel everything, as well as our ability to eat, sleep, and think.

And yet, as remarkable as these moments of loving presence are, it is unbelievably easy to lose sight of how fragile and temporary our love is as we move through the day to day details of maintaining life. I remember well the relentless grind of sporting events, laundry piles, meal preps and cleanups, and homework among my four kids and husband that left me little space to appreciate how much I loved them. At the moments when I would forget how precious they were to me (which happened more frequently than I would like to admit), I would shake myself awake to the gift of them by the simple practice of imagining this moment as the last time. Watching them walking away from me at their elementary school door or, as I do now, at their dorm or an airport, I let myself deeply feel the brief, intense pang of what it would be if I was never to see them again walking away from me or toward me. It always brings me to tears.

I think of this "last time" practice as preparation for the moment when it will be true—when I will not see or hear or feel them again. Cognitively we know that this is true, that grief is our reward for a life well loved, and we resist the experience, even for a moment, thinking it morose to invite those feelings in. But what I have found is that courting my relationship to grief has been the most powerful way for me to expand into a profound physical sensation of gratitude.

Learning how to bring our own full presence into our relationships is the most treasured and valuable thing we have to offer each other. When we recognize that life is not an inexhaustible well, but rather a collection of brief and tender moments, gratitude is the only sane response. The events that matter, that make you who you are—laughing with someone you love, lying awake at night to the sound of someone's rhythmic breathing, the utter sweetness of a small child's hand in yours—these moments and their memories happen only a limited number of times. Recognizing that our days are numbered and being awake to the small acts that are the legacy of our love is time well spent, a life well lived.

I started this book by asking how we become more human, how we learn to feel. I've tried to approach that question from many different angles, but there are no simple instructions. Like all the truest life lessons, learning how to feel our lives deeply is something that nobody else can teach us. It is something we learn by giving ourselves fully to our days, one hour at a time. We learn to feel in each moment that we can bring our full presence to the people we love.

Making sex work, embracing your erotic soul and deepening the intimacy in your life, is both a consequence of deep presence and its gift. Healing our selves in our deepest erotic space can only be a deliberate act, and the doing of it miraculously seems to heal everything else. Tapping in to the courage to know your own deepest sexual thoughts and feelings and offering them with your whole being is both a lifework and a lasting gift that will be long remembered. Seeking to forgive old repressed sexual wounds and willingly exploring your sexuality will also expand your humanity to a new level of freedom, a new level of feeling, and will give back to both you and your partner in ways that will transform the meaning of sexual presence.

And in the moments when I can't access any sense of gratitude at all, I try to remember that my life, my presence in this moment, is the result of thousands of loves. It is true for each one of us. Consider the long line of people who came before you, each with their own story, who loved each other, even if only for a moment of conception. All of that love preceded you, invented you. You are a product of the love that has transpired over thousands of years. One day in the distant future, your energy and your inspiration will contribute to the heart of someone you can't even imagine right now.

The meaning and love that you have the chance to make in your life is the only legacy that will count when your days are over. Open your arms wide to the mystery of intimacy and embody the erotic connections, the surrender to heartbreak of loving and letting go, in every moment you can. Hold nothing back. Feel what it means to live in the pure presence of love.

Appendix

Love Oil

L*ove oils* is my term for natural aphrodisiacs that awaken our arousal mechanism and enhance our sexual experience through their scent and feel. Aphrodisiacs excite the senses and stimulate desire, and they have been used for thousands of years to enhance intimacy. Great lovers through history employed scent to trigger their sexual impulses.

The love oils I've created (and sell at Good Clean Love) are emulsions of fragrant essential oils in a neutral-smelling carrier oil from a plant source. Unlike fake fragrances, which are or contain synthetic chemicals, essential oils are derived directly from plant sources. The chemical molecules in a true essential oil actually change brain chemistry. They intensify both our olfactory and tactile senses. My love oils also do not contain the fixatives found in most commercial fragrances; such fixatives block the interaction between the scent and your body's own natural pheromones. Without fixatives, my love oils respond to individual body chemistry. In other words, love oils let you smell like you. The same oil on you will smell different than on your partner, and with the love oil, your bodies together will create a unique scent, which can act as a bridge between the two of you and create a sensuous mind-body connection.

The love oils that I make use a base of apricot kernel and organic jojoba oils, although any type of nutrient-rich base oil, such as almond or sunflower, could be substituted. The magic of love oil is in the essential oil blends that are added. Sandalwood, cardamom, vetiver, frankincense, and rose are but a few of the dozens of essential oils that have been identified as aphrodisiacs. As individual scents are blended together, they create entirely new, unique aromas.

If you decide to experiment with making your own love oil, please do your homework. I did a lot of research on aromatherapy and the safe use of essential oils before mixing my first love oils and bringing them into my bedroom. Just because essential oils are natural doesn't mean they are harmless. They are complex, powerful substances. Many, such as cinnamon and clove, can be very painful when applied to skin undiluted. Consider consulting a professional aromatherapist to make sure you're not creating a love oil that will do more harm than good.

While love oils can be used in place of a personal lubricant, you should avoid using love oils on genitals when you're also using a latex condom, as oil can quickly break down latex, causing condoms to perforate. Love oils can still be used in the bedroom if you're using a condom—just don't get them on the condom! Use the love oils for foreplay, where they are the most potent, and get a water-based lubricant for penetration.

As I studied the art of mixing love oils, I learned that many of the most ancient erotic essences were more valuable than gold for the sensual response they elicited. The reason for their enduring value became clear to me as I developed and sold love oils: many people told me that the most challenging sexual issue they face is awakening their arousal mechanism, or, in other words, wanting to want sex. This is precisely the magic of love oils: by stimulating the limbic brain through the co-located olfactory system, they give us access to the part of our brain where memory, emotion, and sexuality are processed. (See chapter 6, "Sensation," for more on how scent affects our brains.)

Here are some of the ways that love oils help the art of lovemaking.

Love oils can intentionally awaken the arousal mechanism. Give up the idea that sexual desire is a prerequisite for sex or intimacy. Instead, use love oil to wake up the arousal mechanism in the limbic brain. Pay attention to the scents that turn you on, and choose a love oil that contains those specific scents. Avoid other products that contain the same or similar scents, and use your love oil only in the bedroom or other places where you specifically want to trigger sexual arousal.

Love oils make touch more sensuous. Adding love oil to almost any body part makes it sexy. Truly, every inch of your lover's body—the slopes between inner thigh and hip, the curve of the buttocks, the nape of the neck—is more erogenous when you can effortlessly glide your hand across it. Love oils enhance the physical intrigue of touch, allowing you to explore ranges of pressure and different kinds of touch. The combination of aphrodisiac scent and touch can extend the time you make love.

Love oils open up fantasy. Just as scent can quickly trigger memories, it can also give rise to fantasy stories, and through these stories, we discover the hidden source of our erotic energy. Each of us has fantasies that live deep within us. Once you find a favorite love oil and start to use it in the bedroom, the familiar, alluring scent lets you more easily slip into your erotic stories. Love oils let your imagination loose and ignite the images and erotic potential inside. (For more detail, check out chapter 7, "Fantasy.")

Love oils enhance oral pleasure. Sexuality is driven by oral satisfaction. Adding love oil intensifies the sensory and tactile experience of all kinds of oral sex, from the smallest kiss to deep fellatio. Apply love oil everywhere you kiss your lover—lips, breasts, genitals. (Because my love oils use pure, plant-derived essential oils diluted in plant-derived carrier oils, the small amounts you might ingest during oral lovemaking will not harm you.)

Love oils can make lovemaking last longer. Because they enhance lovemaking in all of the above ways, you can use love oils to extend the space and time between arousal and climactic orgasm. So linger. The longer you spend cultivating your arousal, the more powerful the release will be.

NOTES

EPIGRAPH
From the poem "Breadmaking" in *The Essential Rumi*, trans. Coleman Barks (New York: HarperCollins, 1995), 183–185.

CHAPTER I, FREEDOM
1. According to UNICEF, "While the exact number of girls and women worldwide who have undergone FGM/C remains unknown, at least 200 million girls and women in 30 countries have been subjected to the practice"; "UNICEF Data: Monitoring the Situation of Children and Women," accessed November 9, 2016, http://data.unicef.org/topic/child-protection/ female-genital-mutilation-and-cutting/#.
2. "Sexual Assault and Rape on U.S. College Campuses: Research Roundup," Journalist's Resource, accessed November 9, 2016, journalistsresource.org/studies/society/public-health/sexual-assault-rape-us-college-campuses-research-roundup; David Cantor, Bonnie Fisher, Chibnall Susan, Reanne Townsend, Hyunshik Lee, Carol Bruce, and Gail Thomas, "Report on the AAU Campus Climate Survey on Sexual Assault and Sexual Misconduct," *Westat* (September 21, 2015), accessed November 9, 2016, aau.edu/ uploadedFiles/AAU_Publications/AAU_Reports/Sexual_Assault_ Campus_Survey/Report%20on%20the%20AAU%20Campus%20 Climate%20Survey%20on%20Sexual%20Assault%20and%20 Sexual%20Misconduct.pdf.
3. Melina M. Bersamin et al., "Risky Business: Is There an Association between Casual Sex and Mental Health among Emerging Adults?" *Journal of Sex Research* (2013), accessed November 9, 2016, sethschwartz.info/wp-content/uploads/2010/08/Casual-Sex-and-Well-Being.pdf; John Peterson, Stacey Freedenthal, Christopher Sheldon, and Randy Andersen, "Nonsuicidal Self-Injury in Adolescents," *Psychiatry MMC* 5, no. 11 (2008): 20–26,

accessed November 9, 2016, http://www.ncbi.nlm.nih.gov/pmc/
articles/PMC2695720/.

4. Sam Kashner, "Both Huntress and Prey," *Vanity Fair*
   (November 2014), accessed November 9, 2016, vanityfair.com/
   hollywood/2014/10/jennifer-lawrence-photo-hacking-privacy.
5. Helen E. O'Connell, Kalavampara V. Sanjeevan, and John M.
   Hutson, "Anatomy of the Clitoris," *The Journal of Urology* 174,
   no. 4 (2005): 1189–1195; Helen E. O'Connell, Kalavampara
   V. Sanjeevan, and Abdulmaged Traish, "Anatomy of Female
   Genitalia," *Women's Sexual Function and Dysfunction*, edited by
   Irwin Goldstein, Cindy M. Meston, and Susan Davis (Boca Raton,
   FL: CRC Press, 2005), 105–112.

CHAPTER 2, PLEASURE

1. David G. Blanchflower and Andrew J. Oswald, "Money, Sex, and
   Happiness: An Empirical Study," *The Scandinavian Journal of
   Economics* 106, no. 3 (September 2004): 393–415.
2. Roy J. Levin, "Sexual Activity, Health and Well-being—The
   Beneficial Roles of Coitus and Masturbation," *Sexual and
   Relationship Therapy* 22, no. 1 (2007): 135–148, accessed
   November 9, 2016, http://www.tandfonline.com/doi/
   abs/10.1080/14681990601149197.
3. Susan A. Hall, Rebecca Shackelton, Raymond C. Rosen, and Andre
   B. Araujo, "Sexual Activity, Erectile Dysfunction, and Incident
   Cardiovascular Events," *American Journal of Cardiology* 105, no. 2
   (2010): 192–197; Dean Ornish, *Love and Survival: 8 Pathways to
   Intimacy and Health* (New York: HarperCollins, 1998), 25.
4. George Davey Smith, Stephen Frankel, and John Yarnell, "Sex
   and Death: Are They Related? Findings from the Caerphilly
   Cohort Study," *BMJ: British Medical Journal* 315, no. 7123
   (1997): 1641–1644, accessed November 9, 2016, jstor.org/
   stable/25176559.
5. B. R. Komisaruk and B. Whipple, "The Suppression of Pain by
   Genital Stimulation in Females," *Annual Review of Sex Research* 6
   (1995): 151–186.

6. Stuart Brody, "Blood Pressure Reactivity to Stress Is Better for People Who Recently Had Penile-Vaginal Intercourse Than for People Who Had Other or No Sexual Activity," *Biological Psychology* 71, no. 2 (2006): 214–222, accessed November 9, 2016, https://www.ncbi.nlm.nih.gov/pubmed/15961213.

7. Roy J. Levin, "Sexual Activity, Health and Well-being—the Beneficial Roles of Coitus and Masturbation," 135–148.

8. Debby Herbenick, Michael Reece, Stephanie Sanders, and J. Dennis Fortenberry, "Sexual Behavior in the United States: Results from a National Probability Sample of Men and Women Ages 14–94," *The Journal of Sexual Medicine* 7, no. 5 (2010): 255–265, accessed November 9, 2016, http://www.jsm.jsexmed.org/article/S1743-6095(15)33207-0/abstract.

9. Roy J. Levin, "Sexual Activity, Health and Well-being—The Beneficial Roles of Coitus and Masturbation," 135–148; for findings on role of ejaculation in improving immune system functioning, see P. Haake, T. H. Krueger, M. U. Goebel, K. M. Heberling, U. Hartman, and M. Schedlowski, "Effects of Sexual Arousal on Lymphocyte Subset Circulation and Cytokine Production in Man," *Neuroimmunomodulation* 11 (2004): 293–298; for findings on role of ejaculation in prostate health, see Michael F. Leitzmann, Elizabeth A. Platz, Meir J. Stampfer, Walter C. Willett, and Edward Giovannucci, "Ejaculation Frequency and Subsequent Risk of Prostate Cancer," *The Journal of American Medicine* 291, no. 13 (2004): 1578–1586.

10. "Masters and Johnson (1966, pp. 125–126) reported that a number of their subjects used self-masturbation with the onset of their menstruation to relieve minor to major degrees of dysmenorrhoea. The orgasm induced by the activity 'increased the rate of (blood) flow, reduced pelvic cramping when present and frequently reduced their menstrual associated backaches'"; quoted in Roy J. Levin, "Sexual Activity, Health and Well-Being—The Beneficial Roles of Coitus and Masturbation," 135–148.

11. "Overall, 28 percent of the men and 39 percent of the women said that they were affected by at least one sexual dysfunction."

From the Global Study of Sexual Attitudes and Behaviors Investigators' Group, "Sexual Behavior and Sexual Dysfunctions after 40: The Global Study of Sexual Attitudes and Behaviors," *Urology* 64, no. 5 (2004): 991–997, accessed November 9, 2016, https://www.ncbi.nlm.nih.gov/pubmed/15533492.

12. Elisabeth A. Lloyd, *The Case of the Female Orgasm: Bias in the Science of Evolution* (Cambridge, MA: Harvard University Press, 2005), 36; for evidence that women exposed to lower levels of prenatal androgens are more likely to experience orgasm during sexual intercourse because these women have a smaller distance between their clitoris and urethral meatus, see Elisabeth Lloyd and Kim Wallen, "Female Sexual Arousal: Genital Anatomy and Orgasm in Intercourse," *Hormones and Behavior* 59, no. 5 (May 2011): 780–792.

13. Global Study of Sexual Attitudes and Behaviors Investigators' Group, "Sexual Behavior and Sexual Dysfunctions after 40: The Global Study of Sexual Attitudes and Behaviors."

14. Michael P. Carey and John P. Wincze, *Sexual Dysfunction, Second Edition: A Guide for Assessment and Treatment* (New York: Guilford Press, 2012), 42.

15. Meredith L. Chivers, Michael C. Seto, Martin L. Lalumière, Ellen Laan, and Teresa Grimbos, "Agreement of Self-Reported and Genital Measures of Sexual Arousal in Men and Women: A Meta-Analysis," *Archives of Sexual Behavior* 39, no. 1 (2010): 5–56, accessed November 9, 2016, link.springer.com/article/10.1007/s10508-009-9556-9.

16. Betty Dodson, *Sex for One: The Joy of Self-loving* (New York: Crown Publishing Group, 2012).

17. Martin Portner, "A Key to Orgasm: Some Brain Areas Have to Go Quiet," *Scientific American* (March 1, 2016), accessed November 9, 2016, https://www.scientificamerican.com/article/a-key-to-orgasm-some-brain-areas-have-to-go-quiet/.

18. Jenny Wade, *Transcendent Sex: When Lovemaking Opens the Veil* (New York: Simon & Schuster, 2004), 17.

Dear Sounds True friend,

Since 1985, Sounds True has been sharing spiritua
and resources to help people live more genuine, lo
fulfilling lives. We hope that our programs inspire a
you, enabling you to bring forth your unique voice a
for the benefit of us all.

We would like to invite you to become part of our g
online community by giving you three downloadable
an introduction to the treasure of authors and artists
at Sounds True! To receive these gifts, just flip this c
for details, then visit us at **SoundsTrue.com/Free** ar
your email for instant access.

With love on the journey,

TAMI SIMON   Founder and Publisher, Sounds True

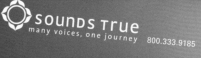

SOUNDS TRUE
many voices, one journey   800.333.9185

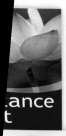
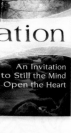
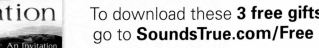
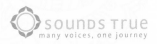

CHAPTER 3, FINDING YOUR NORMAL

1. Alfred C. Kinsey, Wardell B. Pomeroy, and Clyde E. Martin, *Sexual Behavior in the Human Male* (Philadelphia: W. B. Saunders Co., 1948); Alfred C. Kinsey, *Sexual Behavior in the Human Female* (Philadelphia: W. B. Saunders Co., 1953).

2. United Nations Office on Drugs and Crime, *World Drug Report 2011* (p. 144), accessed November 9, 2016, unodc.org/documents/data-and-analysis/WDR2011/World_Drug_Report_2011_ebook.pdf.

3. James A. Simon, Sheryl A. Kingsberg, Brad Shumel, Vladimir Hanes, Miguel Garcia, and Michael Sand, "Efficacy and Safety of Flibanserin in Postmenopausal Women with Hypoactive Sexual Desire Disorder: Results of the SNOWDROP Trial," *Menopause* 21, no. 6 (2014): 633–640.

4. U.S. Food and Drug Administration, "FDA Approves First Treatment for Sexual Desire Disorder: Addyi Approved to Treat Premenopausal Women," press release on August 18, 2015, accessed November 9, 2016, http://www.fda.gov/NewsEvents/Newsroom/PressAnnouncements/ucm458734.htm.

5. Amy Nordrum, "'Female Viagra' Approval: Did Sprout Pharmaceuticals Set a Dangerous Precedent in Earning FDA Go-Ahead for Addyi?" *International Business Times* (August 24, 2015), accessed November 9, 2016, ibtimes.com/female-viagra-approval-did-sprout-pharmaceuticals-set-dangerous-precedent-earning-fda-2063436.

6. Duff Wilson, "Push to Market Pill Stirs Debate on Sexual Desire," *New York Times* (June 16, 2010), accessed November 9, 2016, nytimes.com/2010/06/17/business/17sexpill.html.

7. Emily Nagoski, "The Real Problem with 'Pink Viagra,'" *Los Angeles Times* (August 23, 2015), accessed November 9, 2016, latimes.com/opinion/op-ed/la-oe-0823-nagoski-pink-viagra-20150823-story.html.

8. Martin Portner, "A Key to Orgasm: Some Brain Areas Have to Go Quiet."

9. Ibid.

10. Ibid.

11. Debby Herbenick, Vanessa Schick, Stephanie A. Sanders, Michael Reece, and J. Dennis Fortenberry, "Pain Experienced During Vaginal and Anal Intercourse with Other-Sex Partners: Findings from a Nationally Representative Probability Study in the United States," *The Journal of Sexual Medicine* 12, no. 4 (2015): 1040–1051.

CHAPTER 4, COURAGE

1. Martin Luther King Jr., "Antidotes for Fear," undated sermon, Martin Luther King Jr. Center for Nonviolent Social Change, accessed November 10, 2016, thekingcenter.org/archive/document/antidotes-fear.

CHAPTER 5, CURIOSITY

1. Esther Perel, *Mating in Captivity* (New York: Harper Paperbacks, 2007), 36–37: "I suggest that our ability to tolerate our separateness—and the fundamental insecurity it engenders—is a precondition for maintaining interest and desire in a relationship. Instead of always striving for closeness, I argue that couples may be better off cultivating their separate selves."
2. David Zinczenko, "6 Ways to Get The Sex You Want from Your Man," *Today* (October 15, 2007), accessed November 10, 2016, today.com/id/21270564/ns/today-today_health/t/ways-get-sex-you-want-your-man/#.V7os_K7sdDE.

CHAPTER 6, SENSATION

1. L. Casler, "The Effects of Extra Tactile Stimulation on a Group of Institutionalized Infants," *Genetic Psychology Monographs* 71 (1965): 137–175; Evan L. Adriel and Catharine H. Rankin, "The Importance of Touch in Development," *Pediatric Child Health* 15, no. 3 (2010): 153–156, accessed November 10, 2016, https://www.ncbi.nlm.nih.gov/pmc/articles/PMC2865952/; D. A. Frank, P. E. Klass, F. Earls, and L. Eisenberg, "Infants and Young Children in Orphanages: One View from Pediatrics and Child Psychiatry,"

Pediatrics 97 (1996): 569–578; Evan L. Adriel and Catharine H. Rankin, "The Importance of Touch in Development."

2. B. C. Demirbag and B. Erci, "The Effects of Sleep and Touch Therapy on Symptoms of Fibromyalgia and Depression," *Iran Journal of Public Health* 41, no. 11 (2012): 44–53, accessed November 10, 2016, ncbi.nlm.nih.gov/pmc/articles/PMC3521885/.

3. D. L. Woods, R. F. Craven, and J. Whitney, "The Effect of Therapeutic Touch on Behavioral Symptoms of Persons with Dementia," *Alternative Therapies in Health and Medicine* 11, no. 1 (2005): 66–74.

4. Nicolas Guéguen, "Nonverbal Encouragement of Participation in a Course: The Effect of Touching," *Social Psychology of Education* 7, no. 1 (2004): 89–98, accessed November 10, 2016, link.springer.com/article/10.1023/B:SPOE.0000010691.30834.14.

5. Enid Montague, Ping-yu Chen, Jie Xu, Betty Chewning, and Bruce Barrett, "Nonverbal Interpersonal Interactions in Clinical Encounters and Patient Perceptions of Empathy," *Journal of Participatory Medicine* 5 (2013), accessed November 10, 2016, jopm.org/evidence/research/2013/08/14/nonverbal-interpersonal-interactions-in-clinical-encounters-and-patient-perceptions-of-empathy/.

6. Michael W. Kraus, Cassy Huang, and Dacher Keltner, "Tactile Communication, Cooperation, and Performance: An Ethological Study of the NBA," *Emotion* 10 (2010): 745–749.

7. T. Field, B. Figueiredo, M. Hernandez-Reif, M. Diego, O. Deeds, and A. Ascencio, "Massage Therapy Reduces Pain in Pregnant Women, Alleviates Prenatal Depression in Both Parents and Improves Their Relationships," *Journal of Bodywork and Movement Therapies* 12 (2008): 146–150.

8. Evan L. Adriel and Catharine H. Rankin, "The Importance of Touch in Development."

9. Karen M. Grewen, Susan S. Girdler, Janet Amico, and Kathleen C. Light, "Effects of Partner Support on Resting Oxytocin, Cortisol, Norepinephrine, and Blood Pressure Before and After Warm Partner Contact," *Psychosomatic Medicine* 67 (2005): 531–538.

10. Nadia Christina Oliveira Ramada, Fabiane de Amorim Almeida, and Mariana Lucas da Rocha Cunha, "Therapeutic Touch: Influence on Vital Signs of Newborns," *Einstein (Sao Paolo)* 11, no. 4 (2013), accessed November 10, 2016, scielo.br/scielo.php?pid=S1679-45082013000400003&script=sci_arttext&tlng=en.

11. Dean Ornish, *Love and Survival: 8 Pathways to Intimacy and Health* (New York: HarperCollins, 1998), 139–141.

12. Ross Flom, Douglas Gentile, and Anne Pick, "Infants' Discrimination of Happy and Sad Music," *Infant Behavioral Development* 31(2008): 716–728.

13. Valorie N. Salimpoor, Mitchel Benovoy, Kevin Larcher, Alain Dagher, and Robert J. Zatorre, "Anatomically Distinct Dopamine Release during Anticipation and Experience of Peak Emotion to Music," *Nature Neuroscience* 14 (2010): 257–262, accessed November 10, 2016, nature.com/neuro/journal/v14/n2/full/nn.2726.html; Anne J. Blood and Robert J. Zatorre, "Intensely Pleasureable Responses to Music Correlate with Activity in Brain Regions Implicated in Reward and Emotion," *Proceedings of the National Academy of Sciences of the United States of America* 98 (2001): 11818–11823, accessed November 10, 2016, http://www.pnas.org/content/98/20/11818.long; Ralph Ryback, "Music's Power Explained," *Psychology Today* (January 19, 2016), accessed November 10, 2016, https://www.psychologytoday.com/blog/the-truisms-wellness/201601/music-s-power-explained.

14. Lewis Thomas, *The Youngest Science: Notes of a Medicine-Watcher* (New York: Viking, 1983), 42.

15. Natalie Angier, "The Nose, an Emotional Time Machine," *New York Times* (August 5, 2008), accessed November 10, 2016, nytimes.com/2008/08/05/science/05angier.html.

16. Jordan Gaines Lewis, "Smells Ring Bells: How Smell Triggers Memories and Emotions," *Psychology Today* (January 12, 2015), accessed November 10, 2016, https://www.psychologytoday.com/blog/brain-babble/201501/smells-ring-bells-how-smell-triggers-memories-and-emotions; Gottfried Laboratory, Northwestern University, "Undetectable Smells Influence Human Social Behavior,"

accessed November 10, 2016, labs.feinberg.northwestern.edu/
gottfried/odor_percept_1.html; Claus Wedekind, Thomas Seebeck,
Florence Bettens, and Alexander J. Paepke, "MHC-Dependent
Mate Preferences in Humans," *Proceedings of the Royal Society of
London B: Biological Sciences* 260 (1995): 245–249.

17. On the fitness benefits of heterozygosity, see S. Craig Robertsa,
Anthony C. Little, L. Morris Gosling, David I. Perrett, Vaughan
Carter, Benedict C. Jones, Ian Penton-Voak, and Marion Petrie,
"MHC-Heterozygosity and Human Facial Attractiveness,"
Evolution and Human Behavior 26 (2005): 213–226; on immune
function, see David Haig, "Maternal-Fetal Interactions and
MHC Polymorphism," *Journal of Reproductive Immunology* 35
(1997): 101–109.

18. S. Craig Robertsa, Anthony C. Little, L. Morris Gosling, David
I. Perrett, Vaughan Carter, Benedict C. Jones, Ian Penton-Voak,
and Marion Petrie, "MHC-Heterozygosity and Human Facial
Attractiveness;" Pablo Sandro Carvalho Santos, Juliano Augusto
Schinemann, Juarez Gabardo, and Maria da Graça Bicalho, "New
Evidence That the MHC Influences Odor Perception in Humans: A
Study with 58 Southern Brazilian Students," *Hormones and Behavior*
47 (2005): 384–388.

19. Rachel Herz, *The Scent of Desire: Discovering Our Enigmatic Sense of
Smell* (New York: HarperCollins, 2007), 15–17.

20. Jordan Gaines Lewis, "Smells Ring Bells: How Smell Triggers
Memories and Emotions"; Rachel S. Herz, James Eliassen, Sophia
Beland, and Timothy Souza, "Neuroimaging Evidence for the
Emotional Potency of Odor-Evoked Memory," *Neuropsychologia*
42 (2004): 371–378, accessed November 10, 2016, https://www.
researchgate.net/publication/8963080_Neuroimaging_evidence_
for_the_emotional_potency_of_odor-evoked_memory; Mikiko
Kadohisa, "Effects of Odor on Emotion, with Implications,"
Frontiers in Systems Neuroscience (2013), accessed November 10,
2016, ncbi.nlm.nih.gov/pmc/articles/PMC3794443/#B121.

21. Luisa Demattè, Robert Österbauer, and Charles Spence, "Olfactory Cues Modulate Facial Attractiveness," *Chemical Senses* 32 (2007): 603–610.

22. Jordan Gaines Lewis, "Smells Ring Bells: How Smell Triggers Memories and Emotions"; Rachel Herz, *The Scent of Desire: Discovering Our Enigmatic Sense of Smell*.

23. Sheril Kirshenbaum, *The Science of Kissing: What Our Lips Are Telling Us* (New York: Grand Central Publishing, 2011), 17–18.

24. Mary Oliver, "Low Tide," *Amicus Journal* (Winter 2001): 34.

CHAPTER 7, FANTASY

1. Meredith L. Chivers and J. Michael Bailey, "A Sex Difference in Features That Elicit Genital Response," *Biological Psychology* 70, no. 2 (2005): 115–120, accessed November 10, 2016, https://pdfs.semanticscholar.org/f99d/be15b67312467c2918fab22319f9de983724.pdf.

2. *Fifty Shades of Grey* on Penguin Random House website, accessed November 10, 2016, penguinrandomhouse.com/books/222129/fifty-shades-of-grey-by-e-l-james/9780804172073/.

CHAPTER 8, ATTENTION

1. Mihaly Csikszentmihalyi, *Flow: The Psychology of Optimal Experience* (New York: Harper Perennial, 2008), 66–67.

2. Simone Weil and Joe Bousquet, "L'attention est la forme la plus rare et la plus pure de la générosité," *Correspondence* (Paris: Editions l'Age d'Homme, 1982), 18.

3. Emily Dickinson to Thomas Wentworth Higginson in a letter dated January 1878, *Letters of Emily Dickinson, Volume 1*, edited by Mabel Loomis Todd (North Charleston, SC: CreateSpace, 2015).

FURTHER READING AND RESOURCES

One of my favorite books on my nightstand is *Because It Feels Good: A Woman's Guide to Sexual Pleasure and Satisfaction* (Rodale Books, 2009) by Debby Herbenick. As one of the best-respected sex educators in the country, associate professor at Indiana University, and the associate director of the Center for Sexual Health Promotion at Indiana University, Herbenick has answered thousands of questions from people across the country about everything sexual. *Because It Feels Good* is sexy-smart. Herbenick's years of answering questions and writing columns for national magazines makes her down-to-earth explanations about some of the most blush-worthy aspects of sexuality both approachable and authoritative. Although the book is subtitled *A Woman's Guide,* its wide range of topics would be interesting and of benefit to anyone who loves a woman.

The book is a worthy handbook for anyone's sexual education library because the basic premise is that sex can and should feel good. The author's focus on healthy pleasure and her enlightening discussion of libido and anatomy provide the knowledge that most of us are missing to create more satisfying intimacy. At the back of the book are a plethora of excellent resources for sex and health education; for these alone the book is worth having.

One of my favorite teachers is Tammy Nelson, the author of *Getting the Sex You Want* (Quiver, 2008), which not only has a thorough overview of both male and female erogenous anatomy but also a program of communication skills that makes the previously unspeakable possible for many of us. Although I have not been able to practice all of her suggested exercises, the ones that my husband and I have tried have opened up our ability to ask for what we want and describe what we are thinking in surprising and refreshing ways. This book is one of the best books I've ever read about having conversations about sex.

I also highly recommend *Getting the Love You Want: A Guide for Couples* (Pocket, 2005) by Harville Hendrix, Tammy Nelson's teacher. Hendrix is the creator of Imago Relationship Therapy, which focuses on healing relationships by helping each partner identify the image of the opposite sex they have been unconsciously creating since birth. Hendrix believes that we project these inaccurate images onto our partner as a way of trying to heal old wounds from childhood. As Hendrix shows in this book, when a couple begins to collaboratively witness the faulty images each partner has created of the other, the relationship begins to heal and grow.

Teaching our kids what they really need to know about sex and sexuality is impossible if we ourselves never learned how to have a conversation about sex. In *Sex and Sensibility: The Thinking Parent's Guide to Talking Sense About Sex* (Perseus Publishing, 2001), Deborah M. Roffman, a foremost sex educator (she's so good that both Democrats and Republicans invite her to teach!), provides language grown-ups can use to teach young people about sex. In doing so, she also provides language for grown-ups to articulate to themselves aspects of sexuality they have never been table to talk about before. This has the effect of normalizing a lot of the discomfort many of us grew up with because we never had the words to talk about what we were feeling. It's more than just using correct anatomical names; Roffman really connects the intuitive discoveries we make as we mature about who we are as sexual human beings to the terminology we need to talk with others about those discoveries. Using Roffman's book to teach a kid about sex, you end up teaching yourself. This is a book I go to regularly.

Another great teacher whom aspiring lovers will want to include on their bookshelves is Ian Kerner. His books *She Comes First: The Thinking Man's Guide to Pleasuring a Woman* (William Morrow, 2004) and *Passionista: The Empowered Woman's Guide to Pleasuring a Man* (William Morrow Paperbacks, 2008) (formerly titled *He Comes Next*) are the most intelligent and thoughtful discourses I have ever read on oral sex. Far from merely offering a how-to guide, although there is plenty of that too, his thinking about what oral sex means and how it is experienced for men and women is thought provoking and will challenge your assumptions. *Sex Detox: Recharge Desire, Revitalize Intimacy, Rejuvenate Your Love Life* (HarperCollins, 2009), another of Kerner's books, offers a program for getting out of a sexual rut and starting anew.

Releasing yourself from your fears of sex and sexuality is key for having sex that works. Because many of these fears have been with us since we were children, moving beyond them is not easy and often requires a good guide. *Sexual Intelligence: What We Really Want from Sex and How to Get It* (HarperCollins, 2012) by Marty Klein is one of the best I can recommend. Klein, whose advice manages to be both provocative and grounded in common sense, is a great promoter of openness around sex—in relationships and in society. If you connected with the material in chapter 3 of this book, "Finding Your Normal," you should check out Klein's work. He is the king of normalizing sex.

Finding a language for exploring the exciting experience of letting go and having the courage to change your thinking and habits are the subjects of Vivienne Cass's *The Elusive Orgasm: A Woman's Guide to Why*

She Can't and How She Can Orgasm (Brightfire Press, 2004). In a therapeutic workbook style, which guides the student through rethinking
her relationship to her own sexuality and making the changes necessary to experience it, this book is a great introduction to uncovering
the sexual pleasure that is our birthright.

⚘

Maybe the smartest book I have ever read about how sexual attraction happens and why it is such a powerfully transformative healing
response is Stanley Siegel's *Your Brain on Sex: How Smarter Sex Can
Change Your Life* (Sourcebooks, Inc., 2011). The basic premise is that
our brain is continually working subconsciously to heal us, which
explains what happens in our dream time and in our fantasy time.
Our dreaming brain reconfigures our unresolved emotional issues and
internal conflicts as we sleep in order to bring us peace—or, in the case
of our erotic fantasies, to make pleasure out of pain.

This fantasy-making process happens for us without our conscious
knowledge or participation in early adolescence, as our erotic self
emerges. Whether our emotional issues relate to abandonment, over-
bearing parents, or acute levels of unworthiness, our brain uses those
painful childhood experiences to create a sexual fantasy life that transforms the pain into sexual pleasure. The route is circuitous and rarely
follows any predictable form, which is why in many ways our sexual
fantasies are unique, like our fingerprints, and yet they are also universal, in that we all have them.

One anecdote that Siegel shared with me makes this process clear:
There was a young woman who grew up in an extremely religious
family in which sin and pleasure were synonymous. Years later, she
discovered that her most powerful and unyielding fantasy was to
have sex with her husband while she was dressed up as a nun and her
husband was dressed as a priest. Her husband was happy to oblige
and much pleasure was had, while something deep in her was also
healed. This case simplifies the phenomenon of how her subconscious eroticized early, painful limits into their opposite. Having

consciously made the connection to her past, she played out her fantasy with her husband, and the emotional trauma began to have less and less of a hold on her. Her role-playing also expanded the intimacy she had with her husband.

Some fantasies are not as easily matched to the wounding that happened, and the subconscious selections don't necessarily correspond in a linear fashion. Abandonment issues, for example, can turn into submission or domination fantasies and even translate into common fetishes, because a painful loss can be replaced with a strong erotic association to another seemingly obscure object.

In another of my favorite books, *Women's Anatomy of Arousal: Secret Maps to Buried Pleasure* (Mango Garden Press, 2009), author Sheri Winston (who was a midwife for twenty years) describes the layers of female sexual anatomy as a journey into a sacred temple. She also provides clear, hand-drawn images that show both the separate parts and their relationship to each other. Reflecting on how the world would be different for millions of us had we all been privileged as children to have her compassionate and straightforward anatomy lessons is like imagining a true revolution in self-love.

Winston devotes an entire chapter to understanding the complex physiological causes and effects that transform arousal into orgasm for both women and men. It is a fascinating lesson for both genders to recognize how our arousal mechanisms are similar in capacity but how their different anatomical locations make all the difference in our experience.

One of the books that most significantly informed my own sexual awakening is Rebecca Chalker's *The Clitoral Truth* (Seven Stories Press, 2000). I still remember my own amazement at discovering the complexity and depth of the clitoral system and how that new understanding changed the way I understood everything about my own sexuality. Chalker is a master sex educator and activist, whose in-depth exploration of female anatomy and sexual response cannot help but expand your knowledge of your own body. A must-read for any woman or couple on a pleasure quest.

In *Shameless: How I Ditched the Diet, Got Naked, Found True Pleasure . . . and Somehow Got Home in Time to Cook Dinner* (Rodale, 2011), Pamela Madsen shares her personal journey of sexual exploration with paid body workers in sometimes graphic descriptions but also in prose that is funny, brazen, and bold. The journey itself not only enlivened her marital sex life but also healed her from years of failed diets and body-image issues.

Madsen gives very intimate details, and there were moments when I was troubled reading her story—mostly by the secrets she kept from her husband. But the healing journey was too important to her to abandon, even as she realized that its healing could cost her a great deal of the rest of her life.

Esther Perel is one of the most articulate and thoughtful sex therapists of our time. In *Mating in Captivity: Unlocking Erotic Intelligence* (Harper, 2007), her deeply intuitive perspective on the connections and breakdowns between intimate relationships and sexual intimacy is at once enlightening and transformative. Her book is one of my go-tos when I get lost in my own domestic trials and can't find my way back to the bedroom. While a lot of her wisdom is counterintuitive, it is fresh and true on most every page.

A research study on transcendent, or sacred, sex by Jenny Wade is recorded in her book *Transcendent Sex: When Lovemaking Opens the*

Veil (Simon and Schuster, 2004). Earlier studies suggest that as many as one in twenty individuals have a transcendent experience and that over 80 percent of them keep the experience a secret even from their partners. All of the people in Wade's study had no previous experience or training in transcendent practices, and most had no real language or framework in which to understand their experience.

Interestingly, the variety of experiences was as vast and unique as the survey sample itself. The range of experiences cited in the book cover everything from a shift in space and time, to a sense of electric light-filled bodies, to transformation of self and other, to a sense of timelessness and vast emptiness. All of the experiences carry a transformative recognition of the intersecting paths of spirit and sexuality.

David Schnarch understands more about love and sex in committed relationships than anyone else around. His book *Passionate Marriage: Keeping Love and Intimacy Alive in Committed Relationships* (W. W. Norton & Company, 1997) is commonly referred to as "the modern day Masters and Johnson." It teaches me every time I read it.

For example, he points out that people in the same bed, in the same sexual experience, often have totally different expectations, experiences, and desires. And because it is often hard to find our own words for how we express ourselves in larger ways, he offers descriptions of a few lovemaking styles.

Sexual trance involves focusing on body sensations. This is the kind of sex people enjoy when they want to get out of their head. They prefer little talk during sex, and their sexual experiences have an inward focus on experiencing their own sensuality. Good sex feels like an altered state of consciousness.

Partner engagement is all about the emotional bond between you and your partner. Couples in this space enjoy eyes-open sex and have a lot of affection and romance. This is the kind of sex that romance movies and novels celebrate—sex that is a surrendering to the unity and oneness of the couple experience.

Role-playing is the theater arts of sexual experience. Fantasies enliven and enrich the couple and are shared and acted out freely. At its best, this kind of sex is not about acting; rather, the partners become their roles so completely that the experience frees them from even their own ideas. Orgasms are dramatic and expressive.

Sexual encounters can mix all three of these styles, or a person may be pretty committed to a single approach. If you want to learn more about these distinctions and also about the joys of eyes-open sex, pick up *Passionate Marriage* or any of Schnarch's other books.

Sex that works is not possible without emotional intelligence. For that reason, *Emotional Intelligence* (Bantam, 2005) by Daniel Goleman is a must-read for anyone interested in better understanding how to live in more harmonious relationship with others—and with themselves.

Stan Tatkin's book *Wired for Love: How Understanding Your Partner's Brain and Attachment Style Can Help You Defuse Conflict and Build a Secure Relationship* (New Harbinger Publications, 2012) is where I learned about the importance of the relationship as a container for intimacy. He writes about understanding the conflicts that come up in intimate relationships as impersonal—not about one person being "bad" or "good." Tatkin tells us that conflicts happen because both partners are attached to who they are as individuals and lack information about the container they are trying to grow to hold themselves. For a relationship to survive, it is crucial for both partners to move beyond individual concerns and focus on building the strength of the love vessel that contains them. Just from my own experience, I can attest to how crucial Tatkin's message is for long-term love.

A General Theory of Love (Vintage, 2001) is a beautiful book about the biological basis of love, written by Thomas Lewis, Fari Amini, and Richard Lannon, psychiatry professors at the University of California, San Francisco. Making love the basis of research-based study, the authors explore how love affects us biologically and how we in turn affect culture through our expressions of love. Some of the most riveting insights I have ever read about love are contained in this book.

Another book I highly recommend for both the beauty and concision of the author's insights is *A Natural History of Love* (Vintage, 1995) by Diane Ackerman. Ackerman is an incredible researcher and so articulate in thinking about love and how love functions.

Since scent is our primary sense when it comes to sex, and because it was my gateway to understanding my own arousal mechanism, I can't not mention *The Scent of Desire: Discovering Our Enigmatic Sense of Smell* (Harper Perennial, 2008) by Rachel Herz. In this fascinating book, Herz, a professor at Brown University who studies the psychology of smell, explains the neurobiological basis for why certain things smell so good to us and the implications for sexual attraction.

As much as I love books that anchor love and attraction with scientific research, I also deeply appreciate a more spiritual perspective on the mysteries and power of desire. In *The Soul of Sex: Cultivating Life as an Act of Love* (Harper Perennial, 1999), author Thomas Moore offers such a perspective, exploring the divine origins of human sexuality through myth. He argues that the media's obsession with sex is a symptom of our failure as a culture to weave sex into the whole of life. Good food, friendship, and time in nature give our sexuality a broad and supportive base. By emphasizing the importance of all sensual experience, Moore argues, society can create a public life that is erotic and affirms desire and pleasure.

When we are wholly absorbed in the moment and feel as if we are not separate from what we are doing, we are having an experience Mihaly Csikszentmihalyi calls "flow." His book *Flow: The Psychology of Optimal Experience* (Harper Perennial, 2008) describes the experience and argues for its vital importance to our lives. Without it, he says, we feel bored and disconnected, but when we learn to cultivate it, we enrich our lives and gain priceless insights into ourselves and what matters most to us. Read in the context of sex and love, *Flow* is a fascinating, practical guide to connecting with ourselves and each other.

At its best, erotica can spark our fantasies, awaken our senses, and get us in touch with our inherent sexiness, which makes erotica a must-have for your sexual health library. The trouble is, finding the best erotica can mean wading through a lot of not-so-good and therefore desire-deadening writing. Thankfully there is one press that is consistently publishing some of the best erotica being written today: Cleis Press. If you're new to Cleis's books, check out one of their *Best Women's Erotica* anthologies or browse their catalog online to find the subgenre that most intrigues you.

The first time I learned anything about Tantric practices in bed was right after I was married, when my husband and I were trying to learn how to get our libidos to match up. We studied *Taoist Secrets of Love: Cultivating Male Sexual Energy* by Mantak Chia (Aurora Press, 1984; Michael Winn, collaborator), and slowly, through frustrating rounds of practice, we learned techniques to satisfy both of us. It wasn't until just recently that I was gifted with *Tao Tantric Arts for Women: Cultivating Sexual Energy, Love and Spirit* by Minke deVos (Destiny Books, 2016), which is full of even richer and juicier techniques that will heighten your highest highs sexually.

Both of these books are based in the ancient Taoist secrets of lovemaking. There is so much to learn, and both books are extremely accessible.

Visiting a counselor or therapist can be a great way to get answers to questions you have about sex but just can't ask anyone else. It can also be very helpful at times to work through a rough patch in your relationship by visiting a marriage counselor with your partner. Some of the best organizations for relationship and sexuality counseling out there maintain websites with information about the benefits of different kinds of therapies, as well as links to help you find a therapist in your area. Here are some good places to start:

- American Association for Marriage and Family Therapy (AAMFT), aamft.org, 703-838-9808

- American Association of Sexuality Educators, Counselors, and Therapists (AASECT), aasect.org, 202-449-1099

- Society for Sex Therapy and Research (SSTAR), sstarnet.org, 847-647-8832

The website for the Pelvic Solutions Center has a list of excellent resources for women experiencing pain with sex (pelvicsolutionscenter. com/PatientResources/Links.aspx). There are many different causes for pain with sex, so if this is something you are experiencing, it is important not to give up searching for a solution, even if one particular treatment or therapy does not bring relief.

A wonderful resource for anyone experience vulvodynia—chronic vulvar pain—is the website of the National Vulvodynia Association: nva.org. The NVA is a nonprofit dedicated to educating people and coordinating information about this condition. On its website you'll find a health care provider list, support services, self-help tips, opportunities to participate in research, and much more. The wealth of information on the NVA's site is a reminder to any woman experiencing chronic vulvar pain that she is not alone.

The website Kinsey Confidential (kinseyconfidential.org) was designed to give college-age adults information about sexual health, but it has become the go-to for millions, young and old alike. Thanks to the skillful and concise writing of Debby Herbenick, and backed by some of the most progressive sexual health research performed in the country, Kinsey Confidential is an excellent resource for the most up-to-date and accurate information on just about any sexuality topic you could imagine—and then some.

There are also some great tools on the market that help women locate their pelvic muscles and strengthen these muscles by holding and lifting objects inserted into the vagina.

The Natural Contours Energie Kegel Barbell/Exerciser has been a favorite device for providing both weight resistance and exercise training to strengthen the pubococcygeus muscle (better known as the PC muscle).

I have also been a longtime advocate for feminine exercise balls that have been modeled after Oriental Ben Wa balls. Ben Wa balls are marble-sized balls linked by either a chain or a silk string for easy removal from the vagina. Originally used to enhance intercourse, they are now often used to increase the strength of the pelvic floor muscles. Some advanced Pilates instructors use feminine exercise balls to help their students feel the different pelvic muscle groups as they exercise. For many women, the increasing weight allows them to build up their muscles slowly and steadily.

ACKNOWLEDGMENTS

The one thing that all books have in common is that no one ever really writes them alone. So let me come clean right now: although this book has my name on the cover, I consider myself more of a channel than the author of the work.

This book was born one day at the very beginning of my career as a loveologist and purveyor of love products. I was introduced to Tami Simon, the founder of Sounds True, across a firepit at a hotel in Los Angeles. We talked about the book that I aspired to write and how it would give people access to the power of their own intimate lives. She began following my weekly *Making Love Sustainable* newsletter, where I was learning slowly, week by week, what it means to have sex that works.

Yet the most important meeting that made this book possible happened years later. After writing my blog about sex that works—for fifty-two weeks a year for over eight years—I decided that maybe there was now enough material to make a book. I knew from my previously self-published work that I absolutely needed an editor, and so I posted an ad on Craigslist. To my great surprise, the ad attracted dozens of responses. The most interesting replies came from a man and a woman, both of whom had MFAs from Brown University and had previously published books of their own. My first call was to Brian Conn, whom I quickly learned was unaware that the other candidate, Evelyn Hampton, his girlfriend, had also applied for the position. We agreed to interview all together.

What I most remember about that first meeting was the way that Brian and Evelyn's individual intellectual curiosity so easily mingled with their obvious tenderness for each other. Their respectful consideration made the heavy lifting of my thousands of pages of text easy.

This, combined with the skill and training they brought to the writing, assured me that, yes, one day we would have a book.

By our next meeting, a few weeks later, they had teased out the list of themes that are now the chapters of this book. And with Evelyn's assurance that good editing has more to do with deleting excess language than changing the words that were there, we were off and running.

One day, as we were working on the second or third or fourth revision, Brian asked me this: "What if, instead of picking up a new topic each week, you went back to the end of the previous piece and asked yourself what didn't you share—what more can be uncovered to bring yourself more deeply into your own advice?" This question was profoundly challenging and even life-changing, as it allowed me to slowly gather the courage to tell the whole of the story. So now even those readers who have been following my blog for the last ten years will know me in a more intimate way than I have ever before had the courage to express.

Eventually, through this process of deepening and revising the manuscript, Brian and Evelyn and I arrived back at the beginning again, transformed. I don't think any of us knew just how long a road our writing collaboration would be, but I know that had I not been walking this path with them, this book would never have happened. It belongs to them as much as it does to me.

I was fortunate to convince both Brian and Evelyn to join me at Good Clean Love, and their brilliance now shines on in myriad other ways, growing the company and bringing intimate companionship to my days at work. There are few people who have ever gotten me as deeply and with as much sincerity as Brian and Evelyn, and I am grateful every day for the knowing looks, laughter, and confidence they bring to me.

Meanwhile, my fortuitous meeting with Tami allowed me to befriend Jennifer Brown, the director of acquisitions at Sounds True, who provided the critical early feedback on the manuscript-in-progress and whose patient re-readings allowed the book as it is to emerge. And then I was graced with Amy Rost, one of Sounds True's most gifted editors, who brought clarity and eloquence to the effort. I am grateful beyond words to be included in the illustrious family of authors that makes Sounds True what it is today.

Most especially, I am deeply thankful for my family. Without the container of love that is my family, I wouldn't have known a thing about anything in this book. My marriage is not some storybook love affair; rather, as this book makes clear, it has been the most rewarding challenge of a lifetime—a real-life love affair, filled with the contradictions and growth that real love is for. Gratefully blessed with the alchemical, magical, transformative power of sexual intimacy, my husband and I keep riding out the bumps while raising our children, hopefully into better versions of ourselves.

Intimate lives that make us feel are everything, guaranteeing both the height of joy and the depths of sorrow. Those of us who love the most have the most to lose, but I wouldn't have it any other way.

Feel everything.

INDEX

About the Author

"Loveologist" Wendy Strgar is an award-winning entrepreneur, author, and sexual health educator, whose work has helped thousands of people reclaim their passion and heal their relationships. A pioneer in the organic personal care product industry, she is the founder and CEO of Good Clean Love (goodcleanlove.com), a woman-owned Certified B Corporation (B Corp), or a company publicly committed to being a force for global good. *Sex That Works* is the companion to her first book, *Love That Works*.

Wendy started Good Clean Love in 2003 after hearing from many women about, and experiencing for herself, the painful side effects of using petrochemical-based hygiene products. Today, Good Clean Love's products are sold internationally and endorsed by physicians nationwide for their safety. A recent NIH-funded study found Good Clean Love's line of personal lubricant to be one of the safest products of its class.

Wendy has been writing for ten years at the website Making Love Sustainable (makinglovesustainable.com), tackling the challenging issues of sustaining intimate relationships while increasing the awareness of relevant sexual health issues with an authentic, disarming style and innovative advice. She is also a speaker and workshop leader who gives herself fully to sharing the skills of awakening libido, sustaining loving relationships, and raising positivity consciousness. In addition to featured lectures, she offers workshops for cancer survivors at high schools and universities.

Married for over thirty years, with four adult children, Wendy uses her daily life as the laboratory for her loveology work. For more, please see wendystrgar.com.

About Sounds True

Sounds True is a multimedia publisher whose mission is to inspire and support personal transformation and spiritual awakening. Founded in 1985 and located in Boulder, Colorado, we work with many of the leading spiritual teachers, thinkers, healers, and visionary artists of our time. We strive with every title to preserve the essential "living wisdom" of the author or artist. It is our goal to create products that not only provide information to a reader or listener, but that also embody the quality of a wisdom transmission.

For those seeking genuine transformation, Sounds True is your trusted partner. At SoundsTrue.com you will find a wealth of free resources to support your journey, including exclusive weekly audio interviews, free downloads, interactive learning tools, and other special savings on all our titles.

To learn more, please visit SoundsTrue.com/freegifts or call us toll-free at 800.333.9185.